T0299730

Feminist Perspectives in Medical Family Therapy

Feminist Perspectives in Medical Family Therapy has been co-published simultaneously as *Journal of Feminist Family Therapy*, Volume 15, Numbers 2/3 2003.

Feminist Perspectives in Medical Family Therapy

Anne M. Prouty Lyness
Editor

Feminist Perspectives in Medical Family Therapy has been co-published simultaneously as *Journal of Feminist Family Therapy*, Volume 15, Numbers 2/3 2003.

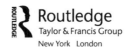

Routledge
Taylor & Francis Group
New York   London

First published by The Haworth Press, Inc.

This edition published 2012 by Routledge

Routledge
Taylor & Francis Group
711 Third Avenue
New York, NY 10017

Routledge
Taylor & Francis Group
27 Church Road
Hove East Sussex BN3 2FA

Feminist Perspectives in Medical Family Therapy has been co-published simultaneously as *Journal of Feminist Family Therapy*™, Volume 15, Numbers 2/3 2003.

Cover design by Lora Wiggins

Library of Congress Cataloging-in-Publication Data

Feminist perspectives in medical family therapy / Anne M. Prouty Lyness, editor.
    p. cm.
"Feminist perspectives in medical family therapy has been co-published simultaneously as Journal of feminist family therapy, Volume 15, Numbers 2/3 2003."
    Includes bibliographical references and index.
    ISBN 0-7890-2546-9 (hard cover : alk. paper) – ISBN 0-7890-2547-7 (soft cover : alk. paper)
1. Family psychotherapy. 2. Family medicine. 3. Feminist theory. I. Lyness, Anne M. Prouty.
    RC488.5.F455 2004
    616.89'156–dc22
                                                          2004002101

Feminist Perspectives in Medical Family Therapy

CONTENTS

REFLECTIONS

ABOUT THE EDITOR

Anne M. Prouty Lyness, PhD, LMFT, is currently a feminist medical family therapist in Fort Collins, Colorado. Previously, she spent a year as Assistant Professor in the master's MFT program at the University of Rhode Island. Prior to that, she taught for five years in the family therapy doctoral program at Virginia Tech, including courses in feminist family therapy, medical family therapy, and family therapy research. Dr. Prouty Lyness is Editor of the *Journal of Feminist Family Therapy*. She has also been active in her state AAMFT divisions, serving in several positions including president, legislative chair, treasurer, and conference chair.

Dr. Prouty Lyness earned her master's degree in marriage and family therapy from the East Carolina MFT program in 1993 and her doctorate from the Purdue MFT program in 1996. She has a lifelong interest in both medicine and feminism, and her writing reflects her clinical and research interests in the mind-body-spirit connection in women's health and the importance of focusing on diversity issues in therapy, training, and research. She has written about feminist internal family systems therapy, college women's help preferences when dealing with disordered eating, the importance of recruiting undergraduates into the profession, and several important aspects of feminist training and supervision. Dr. Prouty Lyness is currently designing research studies investigating mentorship in family therapy training programs and family therapy issues related to women's health and illness.

Preface:
Perspectives in Medical Family Therapy

In recent decades, the influence of gender and human diversity on individuals' and families' experiences of health and illness has become increasingly apparent. Not only do people construct meanings around health and illness differently, but what helps people live healthier lives is also informed by how they experience being in the world. Western medicine, traditionally a man's world full of tools, potions, and procedures, has greatly benefited from an infusion of ideas about the mind-body-spirit connection, previously practiced more often by women caring for loved ones, psychotherapists, religious leaders, and Eastern healers. Because of this "new" biopsychosocial model of healing, women and their families are more often able to obtain care for the entire person (awkward to say "families . . . entire person") when dealing with either everyday or life-threatening illnesses. For example, this biopsychosocial model can explore how family violence might be tied to cancer, how depression affects the immune system, or how cultural beliefs and traditions influence what treatment works better. But this infusion is just beginning in some places, and to varying degrees.

Feminist medical family therapists provide one of those bridges between healthy bodies and healthy relationships. For feminist family therapists, the individual's health issues cannot be understood outside of or separate from one's social systems. We are who we are only when examined within our current contexts, the most important of which are our relationships with others. In this collection of work, several feminists have provided their ideas, research, personal experiences, and suggestions for working with people's bodies, minds, spirits, and relationships simultaneously. Each of these contributions expands the infusion of feminist ideas into our methods of caring for each other as interconnected and diverse beings.

Anne M. Prouty Lyness

[Haworth co-indexing entry note]: "Preface: Perspectives in Medical Family Therapy." Lyness, Anne M. Prouty. Co-published simultaneously in *Journal of Feminist Family Therapy* (The Haworth Press, Inc.) Vol. 15, No. 2/3, 2003, p. xvii and: *Feminist Perspectives in Medical Family Therapy* (ed: Anne M. Prouty Lyness) The Haworth Press, Inc., 2003, p. xiii. Single or multiple copies of this article are available for a fee from The Haworth Document Delivery Service [1-800-HAWORTH, 9:00 a.m. - 5:00 p.m. (EST). E-mail address: docdelivery@haworthpress.com].

xiii

Gender and Biology:
A Recursive Framework
for Clinical Practice

Carmen Knudson-Martin

SUMMARY. This paper applies findings from recent biological research to the historical debate between nurture and nature in the construction of gender differences. Four emerging trends in the biological literature are identified and examined in relation to their implications for how gender is conceptualized and addressed in the practice of marital and family therapy. A multilevel feedback framework for understanding gender differences is proposed and applied to the issue of women's depression. Implications for practice are identified. *[Article copies available for a fee from The Haworth Document Delivery Service: 1-800-HAWORTH. E-mail address: <docdelivery@haworthpress.com> Website: <http://www.Haworth Press.com> © 2003 by The Haworth Press, Inc. All rights reserved.]*

KEYWORDS. Gender, biology, marriage and family therapy, depression, women, feminist psychotherapy, feminist family therapy

---

Carmen Knudson-Martin, PhD, is Professor and Director of Doctoral Programs in MFT in the Department of Counseling and Family Sciences, Loma Linda University, Loma Linda, CA 92350 (E-mail: cknudsonmartin@mft.llu.edu).

[Haworth co-indexing entry note]: "Gender and Biology: A Recursive Framework for Clinical Practice." Knudson-Martin, Carmen. Co-published simultaneously in *Journal of Feminist Family Therapy* (The Haworth Press, Inc.) Vol. 15, No. 2/3, 2003, pp. 1-21; and: *Feminist Perspectives in Medical Family Therapy* (ed: Anne M. Prouty Lyness) The Haworth Press, Inc., 2003, pp. 1-21. Single or multiple copies of this article are available for a fee from The Haworth Document Delivery Service [1-800-HAWORTH, 9:00 a.m. - 5:00 p.m. (EST). E-mail address: docdelivery@haworthpress.com].

Nurture versus nature is a very old debate. Among the most controversial and confusing aspects of the debate are those regarding the essence and origin of gender differences. The relative contributions of biology and social experience in shaping 'masculine' and 'feminine' behavior remain controversial. How one resolves this debate has important political and ethical implications for the practice of marital and family therapy (Knudson-Martin, 1997). The dilemma is especially problematic for feminist practitioners who are concerned that biological explanations of differences tend to reinforce existing gender inequalities.

The feminist concern is that biological explanations for observed differences obscure the impact of social experience on gender. Focusing on differences in how women and men are 'wired' encourages societal and interpersonal inequalities to remain invisible and invites an essentialist perspective, i.e., that differences are natural and cannot be changed (Hare-Mustin, 1987; Knudson-Martin & Mahoney, 1999; Rhode, 1997). Biological explanations suggest that we need to learn to understand these differences and help people accommodate to them in more positive ways. They do not, however, lead us to explore possibilities for changing the differences or ask us to identify and address relational inequalities. Thus, biological explanations tend to be deterministic and perpetuate the status quo.

On the other hand, many feminists have also played a significant role in bringing differences in male and female physiology to light and identifying important gender differences in the meaning, timing, symptoms, and treatment of physical and mental health problems (Anderson & Holder, 1989; Knudson-Martin, 2003). Women are 2-3 times more likely to experience depression and anxiety than men. Onset of schizophrenia is later for women. Women and men respond differently to psychotropic medications and require different dosages for the same body weight (Padgett, 1997). These gender differences have clear physiological implications. Feminist practitioners are concerned that such differences be fully understood and incorporated into models for treatment.

Confounding the nature-nurture debates are ways that ideas and research regarding human biology have been influenced by dominant cultural constructions that emphasize individualism and rationality and use the male body and psyche as the norm (Angier, 1999). Physiological processes related to emotion and affiliation have been less studied and less valued (Taylor, 2002). Thus, biological explanations for behavior have evolved within a narrowed frame for understanding.

In addition, most conventional views of genetic and biological influences have been linear and deterministic (Quartz & Sejnowski, 2002);

that is, that genes and brain structures cause behavior. These explanations leave little room for flexibility, multiple outcomes, and change. Though personal experience, nontraditional medicine, and biopsychosocial approaches to health have suggested a more circular relationship between biology, the person, and the environment, these views tended to be in opposition to the more dominant constructions of human biology and medicine.

This paper focuses on new strands of research emerging simultaneously in the fields of genetics, neuroscience, and endocrinology that fill in many of the gaps in the nurture-nature debate and have major implications for how gender is conceptualized and addressed within the field of marital and family therapy. The author has three objectives:

1. to identify four emergent themes in the biological literature that impact our understanding of human behavior and summarize these findings as they relate to gender,
2. to offer a framework for understanding the dynamic interaction between human physiology, social/interpersonal processes, and gendered traits and behaviors, and
3. to suggest clinical applications of the 'new biology' for marital and family therapy, especially as it relates to gender.

EMERGING THEMES IN BIOLOGICAL RESEARCH

The end of the last century was marked by a flurry of research in brain science and human genetics. According to Steven Quartz and Terrence Sejnowski of the Salk Institute for Biological Sciences, "neuroscientists have learned more about the brain in the last decade than in all previous history" (2002, p. 17). The results of these very technical studies have been so surprising and so significant that a number of highly qualified scientists (such Quartz and Sejnowski) have begun to pull together the interdisciplinary pieces to tell a new story of ourselves as biological and social persons. After reviewing a number of these integrative texts and key research articles cited in them, I identified four interrelated themes that are particularly relevant to our understanding of gender. The first two highlight the roles of emotion and relationship in healthy functioning. The last two suggest a much less deterministic view of biology than commonly believed.

The Importance of Emotion

Emotion has been given a bad rap in Western science. Historically, it has been separated from reason and located in a different part of the brain.

Emotion was 'primitive' and distinct from the more advanced cognitive processes. Emotions, when considered at all, were negative, something that got in the way of rationality. It was assumed that cognition could overcome or override emotion. Associated with the feminine gender, emotion was not trusted, prized, or understood. The new research, however, brings the importance of emotion to the foreground. New studies reveal that emotion and feelings are important components of the ability to make sound judgments (Damasio, 1994; Siegel, 1999). They show a "neuro-biological reality" that emotion and meaning are inseparable (Siegel, p. 159). "Cognition is not as logical as we thought" (LeDoux, 1996, p. 19).

Among the new findings regarding emotion is that it is part of a complete network of communication between the brain and the body (Pert, Ruff, Weber, & Herkenham, 1985; Pert, 1997). Pert's research suggests that three areas previously studied separately–neuroscience (the brain), endocrinology (the glands), and immunology (the spleen, bone marrow and lymph nodes)–are actually joined together by information carriers known as neuropeptides (p. 184). Her work suggests that the mind goes beyond the brain and is in the constant flow of information among the cells. According to Pert, this network of communication represents the "biochemical substrate of emotion" (p. 179). Mind, emotion, and body are inexorably linked. "Emotion," she says, "is at the nexus between matter and mind . . . influencing both" (p. 189). Emotions can thus no longer be thought of as less valid. They are what make the dialogue between the conscious and unconscious processes possible. They are a linking mechanism contributing to an individual's state of health. This means that interventions on the interpersonal and psychological levels can have a direct impact on the body.

According to Damasio (1999), a new generation of neuroscientists and cognitive neuroscientists are focusing on emotion. These studies suggest that emotions assist in reasoning. Rather than a negative influence to be transcended, access to one's emotions not only enhances decision-making, but is prerequisite to it. Studies show that the rational mind may be functioning well (i.e., perception, working memory, etc.), but if emotional reactivity is damaged, a person will not be able to draw on this information to make a good choice (Damasio, 1994). According to Damasio, however, "the biological machinery underlying emotion is not necessarily dependent on consciousness" (1999, p. 43). For example, a controlled study shows that damage to the hippocampus (necessary for the creation of new memories) does not impair the ability of a person to choose the person who 'would be a friend' even though he could not remember previously meeting the person. This new line of understanding emphasizes the positive influence of emotion.

The idea that the brain has a limbic system and that our emotions come out of that place took prominence in the 1950s. The new research shows that emotions involve not only the limbic system, but also the prefrontal cortices and the neural systems that coordinate input from the body. According to LeDoux (1996), emotional feelings involve more brain systems than do thoughts. Emotional information becomes part of the working memory that informs rational thought. In fact, it appears that changes in emotions impact thoughts more than thoughts impact emotions. LeDoux concludes that attempting to change emotions by thinking them away is not likely to work. Though the value of 'feminine' intuitive and emotional skills has historically been discounted, the ability to tap into and respond to emotion is now increasingly recognized as a critical aspect of healthy functioning and an important part of changing human behavior (Atkinson, 1999; Johnson, 2001; Roberts & Koval, 2003).

The Importance of Nurturing Relationships to Health

Considerable research now documents that relationship quality is a significant factor affecting physiology, especially through the impact of the hormones in the stress system (Bower, 1998; Mlot, 1998; Pennisi, 1997). During stress a cascade of hypothalamic, pituitary, and adrenal hormones are released. When the stress becomes chronic (this can be measured by levels of cortisol in the blood or saliva), these hormones shut down the immune cells' responses, muting them and making them less able to defend new invaders (Sternberg, 2001, pp. 111-112). How our body responds, however, depends heavily on our perceptions–the biochemical substrate of emotion identified by Pert (1997)–that link mind and body. In this way, our experiences in our interpersonal environment influence how our bodies respond to stress and directly impact our health.

Though the relationship between positive social support/connection and physical and emotional health has been documented for some time, it continues to be overlooked in diagnosis and treatment. The power of relationship in shaping disease is demonstrated in a study cited by Sternberg (2001, pp. 120-121). In this prospective study, 400 air traffic controllers (a high stress job by anyone's count) were interviewed regarding their perceptions of job and family relationships, and their physical health was assessed. Many of the men experienced depression and anxiety. The factor most predictive of these disorders was the degree of distance and isolation they felt from their employers. Twenty years later, levels of disease including cancer, heart disease, alcoholism, and depression were predicted not by the previous measures in blood, urine, or blood pressure (which was exceptionally high), but by the same psychological factors (isolation) that were related to disease in time one.

According to Sternberg (2001), "we carry our relationships with us in our brain." Stress responses evolve in context of circular interpersonal processes. Less than 50% of our stress responsiveness is in our genes; more than 50% is molded by our environment (Sternberg, p. 148). Whether relationships are a positive or negative impact on our health depends on the quality of the relationship. Different emotions trigger different amounts and types of hormonal responses to stress. Relationships that are stressful and anxiety-producing may increase the ACTH from the pituitary and the cortisol from the adrenal glands. Positive relationships increase oxytocin, a hormone that has a soothing effect and promotes health.

According to Taylor (2002) and her colleagues (Taylor, Klein, Lewis, Gruenewald, Gurung, & Updegraff, 2000), gender bias in studies of stress resulted in an emphasis on 'flight or fight' responses that overlooked 'tend and befriend' responses. Their work suggests that nurturing behavior in response to a stressful situation produces oxytocin in the tending person as well as soothing the other. Thus the attachment-caregiving system plays an important role in regulating stress. While the neuroendocrine circuitry involved may differ somewhat for women and men, Taylor et al. conclude that tending behavior is also stress-reducing for men. Yet, virtually all studies of affiliative behavior have been conducted on women.

Stereotypically gendered behavior appears likely to increase levels of stress. For example, in a study of divorcing couples (Kiecolt-Glaser, Malarkey, Cacioppo, & Glaser, 1994), the confrontive wife faced with an impervious husband showed the greatest increase in stress hormones and decrease in immune function. These authors suggest that the withdrawing spouse puts on a shield that protects against the high stress in this situation. It is the sensitive (usually female) spouse who carries most of the stress. It appears that relationships can be a mixed blessing for women. Women often experience the 'contagion of stress' that is felt when disturbing life events affect those to whom they are close. It is also associated with young children and strains in ongoing relationships (McGrath, Keita, Strickland, & Russo, 1990). Female caregivers experience more stress and less support than male caregivers (Murray, 1996). Yet, friendships and positive intimate relationships remain an important protective factor against stress and illness (Taylor, 2002). Relational mutuality, a balance between the giving and taking, appears to be an important part of relationship quality and contributes to the well-being of both genders (Steil, 1997). Unfortunately, gender differences and inequalities discourage mutual relationships.

Plasticity of the Brain

Adherents of the 'biology is destiny' explanation for gendered behavior are often fond of evolutionary psychology. This view places motives for human behavior in the genes. We behave as we do because of a genetic struggle for survival. In this view "the status quo represents a genetic reality" (Quartz & Sejnowski, 2002, p. 15) that dooms us to behavior preordained by our ancestral past. Men, for example, are more sexuality active than women because it enhanced the ability of their genes to survive. The new biology describes a very different kind of interaction between the brain and the environment (e.g., Buonomano & Merzenich, 1998; Eriksson, Perfilieva, Bjork-Eriksson, Alborn, Nordborg, Peterson, & Gage, 1998; Erzurmlu & Kind, 2001; Ragsdale & Grove, 2001). These studies show a "brain that can detect, and correctly respond to, regular patterns in the environment without your conscious awareness" (Quartz & Sejnowski, 2002, p. 18). The world in which we are immersed "literally helps to shape our brain" (p. 27). The brain and our potential responses are very flexible. This new understanding shifts emphasis away from an evolutionary past.

According to Quartz and Sejnowski (2002), we are programmed to update our behavior in response to rapid social change. As a result of functional magnetic resonance imaging (fMRI) researchers have been able to observe the brain transform itself. Rather than a preset wiring plan, Quartz and Sejnowski describe cortical development as "rough trails of possibility" (p. 40). For example, as blind subjects read words in Braille with their fingers, the "visual" part of their brain, the occipital cortex, lit up. The functional pathways of the "responsive brain" (p. 43) had been changed through interaction. "New challenges throughout life can spur brain cell growth as the brain responds to the demands you put on it" (p. 42). This capacity for the brain to alter its structure and functionality is called plasticity (Buonomano & Merzenich, 1998). The circuits of the brain change as we experience things. Interpersonal experience thus plays an organizing role in determining the development of brain structure in early life and throughout the lifespan (Siegel, 1999).

The organization of the brain develops through layers of experience, making the neocortex increasingly sensitive to the environment. Over time the developmental program relies more and more on the world (Quartz & Sejnowski). Moreover, our responses (our traits) change from one social context to another. This model of human mental life is, thus, "irreducibly social" (p. 57). There is a feedback loop between the social experiences that help shape the developing brain and how we interpret and respond to the social world. One of the most recent discoveries is that the brain's capacity for flexibility is lifelong (Eriksson et al., 1998). In contrast to what was previously believed, it has been discovered that new neurons grow in adult brains in response to new environments. Novelty and new tasks stimulate new growth in the brain.

According to the new brain research, what we do actually shapes the structure and functioning of our brains. We not only do things because our brains enable it, what we do constructs our brains. The effect of the environment and how we respond to it appears to grow stronger over time. That is, infants draw on information already in their brains as a result of genetic structure. But development builds on itself, making the original blueprint more of a rough sketch than a fine-tuned plan (Quartz & Sejnowski, 2002; Taylor, 2002). Our understanding of gender differences must thus be placed in context of the ongoing interaction between the brain, the social environment, and what we do. How we do gender will impact the very structure of the brain itself.

Genetic Indeterminism

One of the most heralded scientific events was the mapping of the human genome. For many people, this was linked with a hope that when we understood our genetic makeup we could know, and perhaps control, our destiny. Yet according to David Baltimore (2001), one of the world's most prominent geneticists and a Nobel Prize winner, one of the unexpected findings of the Genome Project was that the genes could not explain the complexity of our biology. Unless there are a lot more genes than were found, the 34,000 genes that were discovered fall far short of what would be required for programming all the different proteins that make up our bodies. Genes represent the molecular blueprints necessary in mapping the complex proteins that provide for the cell's structure and functions (Lipton, 2001). This includes a transcribing as well as transmitting function (Siegel, 1999). At the same time as the Genome Project has been garnering attention, there has been considerable research documenting the ways in which gene expression (transcription) depends on experience (Siegel, 1999). One of the most important of these findings is that genes cannot turn themselves on or off. Rather, communication mechanisms between the body and the environment activate genes (Nijhout, 1990; Lipton, 1998; Shapiro, 1991; Thaler, 1994). More specifically, according to Lipton, it is the *perception* of the environment that directly controls gene activity.

Though the nucleus of the cell has previously been thought to be the command center for genetic expression of the cell, new research is focusing on the cell membrane. The membrane provides an interface between the cell cytoplasm and the ever-changing environment (Lipton, 1998, 2001). According to Lipton, protein receptor molecules in the cell membrane recognize the environment external to the cell in much the same way that eyes and ears do for the body. This in turn activates effector proteins that selectively "control" cell behavior in coordinating a response to the initiating environmental signal. One of the most interesting findings is that cells not only read their environment, they also make *new* protein receptors to respond to ever-changing environments (Hagmann, 1999; Thaler, 1994). These adaptive responses at the cellular level create new perception proteins in a process representing cellular learning and memory.

Cells innately possess genetic 'blueprints' to create the necessary perception complexes that allow them to survive (Lipton, 2001). However, changes in environments generate the need for new perception complexes. Perception thus plays an important intermediary role between genetics and behavior, both in turning on and off genes and in stimulating genetic change. Genetically programmed perceptions are referred to as instincts. Though instincts are important, humans are more dependent on learned perceptions. Both conscious and unconscious experiences influence perceptive functioning at the cellular level. This cellular learning becomes hardwired into what we know as the brain. And in a recursive process, the functioning of our mind–neural activity dependent on interpersonal experience–produces changes in gene expression (Siegel, 1999). Thus, experience and belief systems directly impact the activity of our genes. According to Lipton (1998), social learning can override 'programmed' genetic behavior.

A recent study by Reiss, Neiderhiser, Hetherington, and Plomin (2000) examined the influence of genetics on adolescent development. They studied pairs of siblings with varying levels of shared genetics (monozygotic twins, natural siblings, step-siblings, etc.) in an effort to sort out what was family influence, what was non-shared environmental influence, and what was genetic influence. Their interpretation of their findings is consistent with the ideas suggested by genetic studies at the cellular level. That is, while genes were clearly influential, genes alone could not explain the complexity of their findings. Reiss and his colleagues postulated a 'relationship code' by which family/environmental factors interact with genes to stimulate responses. Genes, it seems, did not act independently. Whether and how genes were expressed depended both on the environmental context and the individuals' own perceptions of their situations.

These new genetic studies suggest that human 'nature' is much more adaptable than previously thought. Like the brain research, these studies point to a psychological and physical capacity for creative response to a changing environment. Taylor (2002) emphasizes that biologically both sexes have the ability to play almost any social role they choose. Furthermore, what we do changes our physiology. For example, she reports that tending children changes men's hormonal systems. Testosterone levels decrease, allowing other hormones to come into play. At the same time, we are clearly biological persons. The new research is beginning to document how our biology, our social context, and personal experience work hand in hand to create each other.

A MULTILEVEL FEEDBACK FRAMEWORK

Many of the research findings cited above challenge established notions in their fields. The authors are quick to note that they are only beginning to understand the complexity of the processes they are discovering. Though considerable work remains to definitively outline the mechanisms involved, these studies identify important new foci for study and provide new ways to think about human behavior and change. Though studying quite different biological processes, the four strands of research identified here converge in remarkable ways. All focus on interaction between the body and its environment. They begin to explain how perception and response occur at various physiological levels. Emotion and consciousness are identified as key parts of reciprocal, systemic processes linking our bodies and our relationships. They offer a more fluid, dynamic, and relational story regarding our biological and social selves.

Taken together, the four themes identified above suggest that gender differences are an interactive part of reciprocal feedback processes between biological, interpersonal, and sociopolitical influences. This dynamic relationship, conceptually sketched in Figure 1, means that though biology plays a part in shaping gender differences, the interpersonal and sociopolitical processes that also construct gender play a role in how the body responds and shapes itself, even at the neuroendocrine and cellular levels. Explanations of gender differences need to take into account the interaction of each of these dimensions.

Though the specific mechanisms and pathways of influence remain uncharted, this framework helps to explain why biological explanations alone have not been adequate to explain common differences between male and female behavior in areas as diverse as maternal instinct, aggression, sex drive, and mathematical abilities (Kimmel, 2000). For example, understanding physiological responses to stress requires taking into account how stress is influenced by factors external to the body as well as different hormonal interactions for women and men. Social structures, roles, expectations, values, and patterns of privilege and injustice at the sociopolitical level influence how much and which kind of stress one experiences, who will be more supported during times of stress, and how one responds.

On a day-to-day basis, interpersonal processes recreate and maintain gendered social patterns or they revise and defy them. Physiological structure, chemistry, and health are, in turn, impacted and defined. Though stereotypic gender differences in emotional and relational behavior tend to be reinforced and exaggerated at all levels, potential for change on each level is constant, and exceptions to gender typical behavior abound. Emotions and affiliative responses are important parts of the process.

FIGURE 1. A Multilevel Feedback Framework

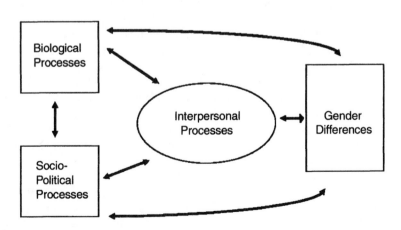

The multilevel feedback framework for gender differences provides a useful guide for thinking about the role of gender in any number of relational, health, and social issues. It encourages us to examine the social and interpersonal context of individual symptoms and calls our attention to ways that gender training and inequalities may be reflected within the body. It invites research that will further define these relationships. Though interventions may be more effective when they address more than one level of influence, this view suggests an important role for interpersonal and societal interventions.

WOMEN'S DEPRESSION: AN EXAMPLE OF THE MULTILEVEL FEEDBACK FRAMEWORK

Depression is one of many gender-related health problems that can benefit from a multilevel lens. I use it here to demonstrate using the feedback framework to examine gender differences. Though depression is an issue that clearly has a biochemical component, neither biology nor social influences alone have been able to explain why women suffer from depression at twice the rate of men (Nolen-Hoeksema, 1987).

Biological Influences

The classical biological understanding of depression is that there is a shortage of neurochemical serotonin secreted by the brain cells (Pert, 1997). To correct this imbalance, antidepressant drugs flood the receptors with serotonin. But the biological story of depression is more complex. Though the biological causes of depression are still far from understood, depression is recognized as part of an interaction between the brain and the hypothalamic-pituitary-adrenal (HPA) axis, that is, the mechanisms for adapting to stress (Sternberg, 2001; Walsh, 1998; Weissman & Olfson, 1995; Young, Midgley, Carlson, & Brown, 2000). Depressed people tend to have higher levels of stress steroids. They are in a chronic state of ACTH (adrenocorticotropic hormone) activation that is stimulated by CRH (cortical-releasing hormone) because the CRH receptors are desensitized and fail to signal that there are sufficient levels of steroid in the blood. The result is a very limited range of behavior. These recursive processes maintain themselves so that the feelings of pain and sadness are retained not only in the brain, but all the way down to the cellular level (Pert, 1997). Researchers are now examining in more depth the mechanisms that create a link between the immune system and mood (Sternberg, 2001). This raises questions regarding both the factors that may subject women to this kind of stress and ways that women's bodies may differentially respond.

There is therefore considerable interest in ways that depression may be related to the female sex hormones (Walsh, 1998; Young et al., 2000). This is because depression is primarily a disorder of women of child-bearing age. Women are twice as likely as men to experience depression and are most at risk around times of hormonal transitions such as puberty, pregnancy, and premenstrual periods. Contrary to popular belief, rates of depression for women decrease following menopause. However, women with a history of depression may also be at risk during perimenopause (Northrup, 2001). Studies examining a link between depression and levels of progesterone and estrogen have mixed results, but do not appear to support a conclusion that depressed women have significantly different hormonal functioning than nondepressed women (Nolen-Hoeksema, 1987; Northrup, 2001; Walsh, 1998). One recent study (Young et al., 2000) reports somewhat lower levels of estradiol among depressed women during the follicular phase only. All other hormonal functioning was similar in depressed and nondepressed women.

Estrogen plays many roles within both female and male bodies. According to Angier (1999) it is not yet well understood. She suggests, however, that it is important to recognize that estrogen is a facilitative hormone. It does not cause particular emotions, but may impact the ones that are present. It permits, but does not create, emoting. Thus it seems likely that understanding what happens to women physiologically when they are depressed is related in some way to the interaction between their biological processes and the emotions and stresses in their lives.

Sociopolitical Factors

Risk for depression is not evenly distributed among the female population. Depressive symptoms are negatively correlated with education and income (Lennon, 1996). White women have fewer symptoms than women of color. Hispanic women have the highest levels of symptoms (Lennon, 1996). Women who have children and live in poverty are more likely than other women to experience depression (Belle, 1990). Women are also frequent victims of violence and sexual abuse. These experiences dramatically increase vulnerability to depression (Harris & Landis, 1997; McGrath et al., 1990).

Women's depressive symptoms have been associated with cultural proscriptions that discourage women from holding or showing power and inhibit the expression of anger (Anderson & Holder, 1989; Kaplan, 1991). Women have historically been taught to hide their strengths and develop indirect influence strategies. They have been encouraged to accommodate to others and to doubt the appropriateness of their own desires or actions. Though ideas about gender are changing, the gendered styles of behaving live on. Sometimes women seek and maintain relationships at the expense of their own well-being. Women's 'passive' responses to depression may perpetuate depressive symptoms (Nolen-Hoeksema, 1987; Walsh, 1998).

Women are influenced by a variety of contradictory pulls from society. Despite their active participation in the work force, women remain the primary caregivers and kin-keepers. They are judged psychologically or professionally deficient when they 'focus too much' on others, but are held accountable for the health and well-being of their families. They are expected to calm and soothe men and to ensure the safety and self-esteem of their children, but they are criticized for being 'over-involved' or 'controlling.' Though some women thrive despite these contradictory pulls, depressive symptoms may also be understood as normal responses to situations with seemingly impossible demands and little recognition (Knudson-Martin, 2001).

Women's social roles have been identified as a major factor contributing to depression (Lennon, 1996; McGrath et al., 1990; Nolen-Hoeksema, 1987). The relationships between depression and women's roles, however, are complex. The women most at risk are single mothers who do not have access to reliable child care. As a group, married women who work outside the home fare better than women who do not. But this depends in part upon the woman's preferences and is strongly influenced by whether her partner shares household and child care tasks (Lennon, 1996; McGrath et al., 1990). Thus, risk for depression must clearly be placed in context of societal patterns of gender, socioeconomic, and racial inequalities. Policies designed to reduce symptoms of depression in women must include efforts to reduce poverty, increase access to child care, and encourage men's involvement in family life (Lennon, 1996).

Interpersonal Factors

Depression in women is highly associated with relationship distress. As suggested by the second theme in this paper (The Importance of Nurturing Relationships to Health), whether relationships serve a protective function or increase the risk depends on the quality of the relationship. The sociopolitical factors addressed above directly impact the quality of interpersonal relationships. Historical socialization patterns tend to perpetuate gender inequality. These patterns easily slip into couple relationships, even when it is not the couple's intention (Knudson-Martin & Mahoney, 1999). Women end up carrying a disproportionate share of the relationship loads, especially in single-parent and dual-earner households. These relationship inequalities are directly related to risk for depression (Lennon, 1996; McGrath et al., 1990).

There is an apparent relationship between perceptions of power in interpersonal relationships and depressive symptoms (Steil, 1997). Steil defines power as the ability to influence important decisions and to get others to do what they otherwise would not. Her analysis of the link between this kind of interpersonal power and fewer depressive symptoms identifies several contributing factors. For example, when persons of either sex perceive power within the relationship, they use direct influence strategies in interpersonal communication. The use of direct strategies is related to higher levels of intimacy and relationship satisfaction for both women and men. Steil concludes that equal power makes intimacy possible. Persons reporting less power are more likely to report depressed feelings. The availability of intimacy is associated with fewer symptoms for men and women. Women, however, are less likely to report this kind of positive experience than men.

A number of studies have shown that the quality of a 'confidante relationship,' that is, a close attachment figure to whom one can tell one's troubles, is associated with psychological health (Romans, 1998). When the relationship is supportive and affirming, health is enhanced and the risk of depression minimized. For women, this relationship may be with their partners, but may also be found with a female friend. On the other hand, partners that are critical or emotionally or physically abusive increase risk (Romans, 1998). A number of researchers are now trying to explain the physiological underpinnings of these various kinds of attachment relationships. Though a number of neurochemical processes are being studied, oxytocin and vasopressin appear to be important contributors to the biochemical processes of attachment and its relationship to health (Quartz & Sejnowski, 2002; Romans, 1998; Sternberg, 2001; Taylor, 2002).

Recursive Processes

The multilevel feedback framework emphasizes the recursive ways in which biological, interpersonal, and sociopolitical processes reinforce each other. Instead of looking for 'the' cause of depression, we will seek to understand the interactive mechanisms that maintain it. Though we do not yet have a great deal of information regarding how the interactions across levels play out, a possible explanation of gender differences in rates of depression based on the 'new biology' may be something like the following.

Possible genetic predisposition toward depression and biologic contributions of the female sex hormones will be translated and activated by her experience in her environment. Living in context of a culture that disproportionately disempowers women impacts her emotional experience. This experience is perceived at the cellular level and becomes part of the flow of information between the brain, the endocrine system, and the immune system. Biochemical, cognitive, and behavioral responses to her situation are impacted by and stimulate an interacting cascade of hormones. At the same time, experience helps to shape the neural pathways that are being constructed in her brain on an ongoing basis. Continued societal and interpersonal experience reinforce or change her perceptions on both conscious and unconscious levels and impact hormonal responses to stress and her perceptions of them. The quality of her ongoing interpersonal relationships plays an important role in her ongoing experience of stress and risk of depression.

In the above scenario, women who lack economic and social supports are most at risk. Biological processes are created and maintained through an interaction between genetic material and day to day experience. These biological structures and processes, in turn, impact how new experience is perceived and translated back into the body. Women who do not feel free to express themselves directly are likely to be especially vulnerable. Treatment that does not address underlying power issues may be ineffective in the long-term. On the other hand, once established, the biological mechanisms supporting depression will mean that change may require time, persistence, support and intervention at multiple levels.

The new themes in biology identified in this article encourage the study of interaction and recursive processes. They bring rays of hope that research and treatment regarding illness, health, and disease will move beyond a linear model of causality that sometimes seems to begin and end with biology. This is particularly relevant to the understanding of gender influences and how we address them. It is not useful to create a duality between biological and social influences on behavior. We do not have to abandon an interest in biological processes to give up the idea that if gender differences have biological components, these differences are "natural" and cannot be changed.

CLINICAL IMPLICATIONS

Marital and family therapy is part of the interactive processes linking body, relationship, and society. The 'new' biology suggests that social and interpersonal processes limit options for both women and men in ways that are not biologically mandated, but may be biologically influenced and sustained. Since stereotypic gender differences are associated with relationship distress (Gottman, 1994), discourage intimacy (Steil, 1997), and contribute to mental health problems (Knudson-Martin, 2003), clinicians are invited to approach gender differences with expectations that gender differences, like our brains and cells, are fluid and flexible.

Traditional differences between women and men have been shaped in context of societal and relationship models based on power differences between women and men. Though gender ideals are considerably more egalitarian today, recursive relational processes and societal structures continue to impact women and men in ways beyond conscious awareness. Women, for example, are still more likely to accommodate in their relationships than men (Walker, 1996; Zvonkovic, Greaves, Schmeige, & Hall, 1996). It is important, therefore, that therapists raise their consciousness about ways that we can avoid inadvertently perpetuating these patterns and position ourselves to take active roles in helping our clients revise them (Knudson-Martin & Mahoney, 1999).

Many models for marital and family therapy do not include attention to gender and power; others over-emphasize and reinforce stereotypic gender differences. The suggestions that follow make a case for many common feminist practices. They are designed to encourage women and men to move beyond the limitations of old gender frameworks and, at the same time, see this work as part of biologic processes. They may be integrated within most MFT models.

1. *Frame gender differences as 'habits' or 'choices' rather than 'instincts' or 'natures.'* This will encourage clients and therapists alike to be open to the possibilities that some of these patterns may be changed.
2. *Explore how clients' gendered roles or behaviors came to be.* When we ask, for example, how a couple decided that she would organize her time around his schedule, hidden cultural assumptions are made visible and clients have more options for how they choose to pattern their lives.
3. *Assume that emotional expression and attending skills are valuable and can be developed by both men and women.* Without con-

scious attention to validating these skills, they are easily over-looked. When it is assumed that they are important and available to both women and men, we are more likely to help clients of either sex develop and value them.

4. *Support clients as they consider and devise new (nongender traditional) responses to their issues.* Breaking free of old gender patterns can raise anxiety at first. Also, neural networks in the brain must reorganize themselves. Part of our role is to help clients manage and persist as new ways of behaving become a part of our bodily experience.

5. *Recognize and make visible ways that hidden gender inequalities play out in clients' lives.* Most clinicians recognize and deal with instances of overt power dynamics such as spouse abuse. It is also important to recognize how the more hidden aspects of gendered power differences may be impacting symptoms. These can easily remain invisible because they seem 'so natural.' When we help clients recognize these patterns, they have more choices. For example, a husband who was in the habit of listening to his wife 'when he thinks it's important' may decide that he doesn't want to perpetuate hidden power in this way.

6. *Create a language for the use of psychotropic medications that places them as part of multilevel processes of change.* When medications are framed as facilitators of change, rather than the cause of change, clients are empowered. They can take an active role in shaping interpersonal patterns and responses to messages from the larger society that are health-promoting. Whether or not medications are part of the treatment, clients can benefit from education regarding how our brains, bodies, and relationships work together to influence our health.

CONCLUSION

Empowering women is a major goal of feminist practice. For family therapists this goal occurs in context of work that emphasizes the link between interpersonal processes, well-being, and gender. It is not separate from our work with men. Another important goal is thus to free both women and men from the limiting constraints of traditional gender processes. But when gendered patterns of behavior are labeled as 'biological,' our ability to impact gender patterns is more difficult. Feminist goals sometimes can seem at odds with nature. The biological research addressed in this article is very helpful in closing this gap. Research is beginning to identify the mechanisms that link body, mind, and relationships in a web of recursive processes.

Family therapists already work from a relational framework that emphasizes the impact of context on individuals. The emerging biological research provides new evidence and explanations for how this happens and helps make visible the ways gender and biology co-create each other. The challenge to feminist clinicians and researchers in family therapy is to build on this emerging framework, to identify models and methods that work more effectively because our understanding is deeper and more integrated across disciplines.

REFERENCES

Anderson, C., & Holder, D. (1989). Women and serious mental disorders. In M. McGoldrick, C. Anderson, & F. Walsh (Eds.), *Women in families: A framework for family therapy* (pp. 381-405). New York: Norton.

Angier, N. (1999). *Woman: An intimate geography.* New York: Random House.

Atkinson, B. (1998). Pragmatic/experiential therapy for couples. *Journal of Systemic Therapies, 17,* 18-35.

Baltimore, D. (2001). Our genome unveiled. *Nature, 409,* 814-816.

Belle, D. (1990). Poverty and women's mental health. *American Psychologist, 45,* 385-389.

Bower, B. (1998). Healthy functioning takes social cues. *Science News, 153,* 391.

Buonomano, D. V., & Merzenich, M. M. (1998). Cortical plasticity: From synapses to maps. *Annual Review of Neuroscience, 21,* 149-186.

Damasio, A. (1994). *Descartes' error: Emotion, reason, and the human brain.* New York: Harper Collins.

Damasio, A. (1999). *The feeling of what happens: Body and emotion in the making of consciousness.* New York: Harcourt.

Eriksson, P. S., Perfilieva, E., Bjork-Eriksson, T., Alborn, A. M., Nordborg, C., Peterson, D. A., & Gage, F. H. (1998). Neurogenesis in the adult human hippocampus. *Nature Medicine, 4,* 1313-1317.

Erzurmlu, R. S., & Kind, P. C. (2001). Neural activity: Sculptor of "barrels" in the neocortex. *Trends in Neurosciences, 24,* 589-95.

Gottman, J. M. (1994). *Why relationships succeed or fail.* New York: Simon & Schuster.

Hagmann, M. (1999). How chromatin changes its shape. *Science, 285,* 1201-1203.

Hare-Mustin, R. (1987). The problem of gender in family therapy theory. *Family Process, 26,* 15-27.

Harris, M., & Landis, C. (1997). *Sexual abuse in the lives of women diagnosed with serious mental illness.* Newark, NJ: Harwood Academic Publishers.

Johnson, S. (2001). Emotion in family therapy. Presentation at the annual conference of the American Association for Marital and Family Therapy. Nashville, TN, October.

Kaplan, A. (1991). The "self-in-relation": Implications for depression in women. In J. Dorgan, A. Kaplan, J. Miller, I. Stiver, & J. Surrey (Eds.), *Women's growth in connection* (pp. 206-222). New York: Guilford.

Kiecolt-Glaser, J., Malarkey, W., Cacioppo, J., & Glaser, J. (1994). Stressful personal relationships: Immune and endocrine function. In R. Glaser & J. Kiecolt-Glaser (Eds.), *The handbook of human stress and immunity* (pp. 321-339). San Diego: Academic Press.

Kimmel, M. (2000). *The gendered society.* New York: Oxford University.

Knudson-Martin, C. (1997). The politics of gender in family therapy. *Journal of Marital and Family Therapy, 23,* 421-437.

Knudson-Martin, C. (2001). Women and mental health: A feminist family systems approach. In M. MacFarlane (Ed.), *Family therapy and mental health: Innovations in theory and practice* (pp. 331-359). New York: Haworth.

Knudson-Martin, C. (2003). Avoiding gender bias in mental health treatment. *Journal of Family Psychotherapy, 14*(3), 45-66.

Knudson-Martin, C., & Mahoney, A. (1999). Beyond different worlds: A "postgender" approach to relational development. *Family Process, 38,* 325-340.

LeDoux, J. (1996). *The emotional brain.* New York: Simon & Schuster.

Lennon, M. C. (1996). Depression and self-esteem among women. In M. Falik & K. S. Collins (Eds.), *Women's health: The commonwealth fund survey* (pp. 207-236). Baltimore: The Johns Hopkins University.

Lipton, B. H. (1998). Nature, nurture, and the power of love. *Journal of Prenatal and Perinatal Psychology and Health, 13,* 3-10.

Lipton, B. (2001). Nature, nurture, and development. Retrieved October 27, 2002, from http://spiritcrossing.com/lipton/nature.shtm

McGrath, E., Keita, G., Strickland, B., & Russo, N. (1990). *Women and depression: Risk factors and treatment issues.* Washington, D.C.: American Psychological Association.

Mlot, C. (1998). Probing the biology of emotion. *Science, 280,* 1005-1007.

Murray, S. (1996). "We all love Charles": Men in child care and the social construction of gender. *Gender & Society, 10,* 368-385.

Nijhout, H. F. (1990). Metaphors and the role of genes in development. *BioEssays, 12,* 441-446.

Nolen-Hoeksema, S. (1987). Sex differences in unipolar depression: Evidence and theory. *Psychological Bulletin, 101,* 259-282.

Northrup, C. (2001). *The wisdom of menopause.* New York: Bantam Books.

Padgett, D. (1997). Women's mental health: Some directions for research. *American Journal of Orthopsychiatry, 67,* 522-534.

Pennisi, E. (1997). Tracing molecules that make the brain-body connection. *Science, 275,* 930-931.

Pert, C. (1997). *Molecules of emotion.* New York: Scribner.

Pert, C., Ruff, M., Weber, R., & Herkenham, M. (1985). Neuropeptides and their receptors: A psychosomatic network. *Journal of Immunology, 135,* 820s-826s.

Quartz, S., & Sejnowski, T. (2002). *Liars, lovers, and heroes: What the new brain science reveals about how we become who we are.* New York: Harper Collins.

Ragsdale, C. W., & Grove, E. A. (2001). Patterning the mammalian cerebral cortex. *Current Opinion in Neurobiology, 11*, 50-58.

Reiss, D., Neiderhiser, Hetherington, M., & Plomin, R. (2000). *The relationship code: Deciphering genetic and social influences on adolescent development.* Cambridge, MA: Harvard.

Rhode, D. (1997). *Speaking of sex: The denial of gender inequality.* Cambridge, MA: Harvard.

Roberts, T., & Koval, J. (2003). Applying brain research to couple therapy: Emotional restructuring. *Journal of Couple & Relationship Therapy 2*(1), 1-14.

Romans, S. (1998). Women and social relatedness. In S. Romans (Ed.), *Folding back the shadows: A perspective on women's mental health* (pp. 97-114). Dunedin, New Zealand: University of Otago.

Shapiro, J. A. (1991). Genomes as smart systems. *Genetica, 84,* 3-4.

Siegel, D. (1999). *The developing mind: How relationships and the brain interact to shape who we are.* New York: Guilford.

Steil, J. (1997). *Marital equality: Its relationship to the well-being of husbands and wives.* Newbury Park, CA: Sage.

Sternberg, E. (2001). *The balance within: The science connecting health and emotions.* New York: W. H. Freeman.

Taylor, S. (2002). *The tending instinct: How nurturing is essential to who we are and how we live.* New York: Holt.

Taylor, S., Klein, L. C., Lewis, B., Gruenewald, T., Gurung, R., & Updegraff, J. (2000). Behavioral responses to stress in females: Tend-and-befriend, not fight-or-flight. *Psychological Review, 107,* 411-429.

Thaler, D. S. (1994). The evolution of genetic intelligence. *Science, 264,* 224-225.

Walker, A. (1996). Couples watching television: Gender, power, and the remote control. *Journal of Marriage and Family, 58,* 813-824.

Walsh, A. (1998). Women and mood: Biological considerations. In S. Romans (Ed.), *Folding back the shadows: A perspective on women's mental health* (pp. 165-176). Dunedin, New Zealand: University of Otago.

Weissman, M., & Olfson, M. (1995). Depression in women: Implications for health care research. *Science, 269,* 799-801

Young, E., Midgley, R., Carlson, N., & Brown, M. (2000). Alteration in the hypothalmic-pituitary-ovarian axis in depressed women. *Archives of General Psychiatry, 57,* 1157-1162.

Zvonkovic, A., Greaves, K., Schmeige, C., & Hall, L. (1996). The marital construction of gender through work and family decisions. *Journal of Marriage and Family, 58,* 91-100.

Power and Gender Issues
from the Voices
of Medical Family Therapists

Gary H. Bischof
Monica L. Lieser
Carolyn G. Taratuta
Adriana D. Fox

SUMMARY. Explicit attention to issues of power and gender has been quite limited in the medical family therapy literature. A previous qualitative inquiry on which this current study is based revealed the influence of these issues, even though participants were not asked explicitly about power or gender. This study qualitatively analyzed interviews with 13 family therapists working in nonacademic medical settings for evidence

---

Gary H. Bischof, PhD, is Assistant Professor and Program Director of the Marriage and Family Therapy Master's program in the Department of Counselor Education and Counseling Psychology at Western Michigan University, 3102 Sangren Hall, Kalamazoo, MI 49008 (E-mail: gary.bischof@wmich.edu).

Monica L. Lieser, BS, is a master's student in Marriage and Family Therapy, Department of Counselor Education and Counseling Psychology, Western Michigan University, and a therapy intern with Family Therapy Connections at the Collaborative Health Care Center, Lansing, MI.

Carolyn G. Taratuta, RN, BSN, is a master's student, Department of Counselor Education and Counseling Psychology, Western Michigan University, and a staff nurse on the Cardiac Progressive Care Unit, Munson Medical Center, Traverse City, MI.

Adriana D. Fox, MA, is a doctoral student in Counselor Education, Department of Counselor Education and Counseling Psychology, Western Michigan University.

[Haworth co-indexing entry note]: "Power and Gender Issues from the Voices of Medical Family Therapists." Bischof, Gary H. et al. Co-published simultaneously in *Journal of Feminist Family Therapy* (The Haworth Press, Inc.) Vol. 15, No. 2/3, 2003, pp. 23-54; and: *Feminist Perspectives in Medical Family Therapy* (ed: Anne M. Prouty Lyness) The Haworth Press, Inc., 2003, pp. 23-54. Single or multiple copies of this article are available for a fee from The Haworth Document Delivery Service [1-800-HAWORTH, 9:00 a.m. - 5:00 p.m. (EST). E-mail address: docdelivery@haworthpress.com].

http://www.haworthpress.com/web/JFFT
Digital Object Identifier: 10.1300/J086v15n02_02

of power and gender issues in their experiences collaborating with health care providers. Power concerns voiced by study participants included feeling one-down, unidirectional accommodation, reimbursement problems, professional identity issues, and practical matters having to do with office space, prescribing medication, and confidentiality. Participants further reported influencing medical setting staff and being viewed by some of their medical collaborators as threatening. Gender issues were evident in the lack of males doing this work in nonacademic settings, feminine role expectations in the "male" medical culture, the unique role of female sex therapists, and in the additional roles and gender-informed career decisions of the participants. Suggestions for continued attention to these issues in the growing field of medical family therapy are offered. *[Article copies available for a fee from The Haworth Document Delivery Service: 1-800-HAWORTH. E-mail address: <docdelivery@haworthpress.com> Website: <http://www.HaworthPress.com> © 2003 by The Haworth Press, Inc. All rights reserved.]*

KEYWORDS. Medical family therapy, collaboration, power, gender, qualitative research, behavioral health care

In this selective review of the literature, we summarize some of the key issues related to gender and power in medical settings. A limited amount of literature in the medical family therapy field explicitly discusses power or hierarchy, yet gender issues in the collaborative relationship between the family therapist and health care providers are virtually ignored. The terms power or gender, for example, do not appear in the index of one of the foundational texts in the field–*Medical Family Therapy*–other than mentioning gender issues related to patient health, marriages, and child-rearing, but ignoring direct mention of gender in collaboration itself (McDaniel, Hepworth, & Doherty, 1992). Given this limited direct attention, we draw from literature in related fields such as nursing and psychology that have also attempted to find a place in the overall medical culture.

One overt discussion of power does appear in a prominent book in the medical family therapy field. In *Models of Collaboration*, the authors identify three ways issues of marginality and power exist for the collaborating therapist (Seaburn, Lorenz, Gunn, Gawinski, & Mauksch, 1996). First, many medical family therapists may feel marginalized from their own profession. There may be no other mental health professionals in their setting, and other family therapists may not understand why they would want to work in a medical setting. Second, the family therapist working in a medical setting will likely feel marginal in relationship to the field of medicine, with its own language and culture that differs from that of the mental health field. At times, the medical family therapist may feel very isolated. Third, the feeling of being marginalized can reflect the relationship that exists between the professional fields themselves. Family therapy has been characterized as a field on the margin of psychiatry (Shields, Wynne, McDaniel, & Gawinski, 1994). Family medicine, the primary care medical specialty that has been at the forefront in efforts to collaborate with family therapy, has faced similar difficulties in being viewed as marginal or less desirable among the various medical specialties. The overall effect of marginalization on the mental health professional can be a feeling of isolation, identity confusion, and limited power in decision making.

Power issues are a key consideration in determining the level of collaboration. Doherty and colleagues (Doherty, 1995; Doherty, McDaniel, & Baird, 1996) developed a model of five levels of collaborative care. These levels offer choices and options about how to work together and describe the depth and sophistication of collaborative health care. The levels refer to the extent to which collaboration occurs and to the capacity for collaboration in a given health setting as a whole. The five levels are hierarchical, with greater levels of systemic collaboration and integration at the higher levels. How power issues are dealt with and whether they are directly addressed among the members of the collaborative team are some of the key criteria used to establish the level of collaboration. These levels range from Level 1: Minimal collaboration, where mental health and other health care professionals work in separate facilities, there is little interaction between them, and power issues are not directly addressed, to Level 5: Close collaboration in a fully integrated system in which mental health and other health care professionals share the same sites, vision, and systems in a seamless web of biopsychosocial services, regular collaborative team meetings are held to discuss both patient issues and team collaboration issues, and there is a self-conscious effort to balance power and influence among the professionals according to their roles and areas of expertise. This fifth level of collaboration is rarely seen, but is something to which healthcare professionals can aspire.

Other health care team members besides therapists have faced the hierarchy and patriarchy of medicine. Nursing has long struggled with issues of power and gender. Campbell-Heider and Pollock (1987) suggest that cultural stereotypes have contributed to the perpetuation of hierarchical relations between the two sexes. This theme plays out in the physician-nurse relationship. The nursing profession has been frequently identified as being performed primarily by women. Over the years, this role-stereotyping has preserved the mentality that nurses are to be viewed as physicians' subordinates. Sweet and Norman (1995), taking a historical perspective, indicate that gender divisions have been significant in the relationships between nurses and doctors. In the 19th century, the doctor-nurse relationship was compared with the relationship between that of husband and wife in the family, where the wife takes on a subordinate role. However, in the last 30 years, the feminist and self-help movements have empowered many women; likewise, nurse-practitioners have found a more authoritative voice in the health care field and have been successful at defining their professional identity, separate from that of the field of medicine (Candib, 1995).

Regarding the issue of power, the professional literature portrays the medical doctor as being omnipotent, ultimately responsible for the welfare of the patient. The role of nurse in this relationship has been minimized, viewed as "physician extenders or helpers, under the authority of a physician team leader" (Campbell-Heider & Pollock, 1987, p. 421). A similar idea has been emphasized regarding the physician-psychologist relationship. Bernard (1992) suggests that "in most hospitals, administrators and physicians, not psychologists, are the policymakers and the power holders" (p. 77). Good (1992) describes some of the obstacles that new psychologists face while working in a hospital setting, which are similar to those noted above regarding the marginalization of medical family therapists. The medical culture is clear about making the distinction between psychologists and "real doctors." In a similar tone, he discusses the challenges that psychologists encounter in an attempt to develop working relationships with physicians, and concludes that psychologists working in a hospital setting are often treated as "second-class professionals" (p. 73). This may be magnified for the family therapist, whose stature in the mental health field is generally viewed as less than that of psychologists, who are more universally reimbursed for their services.

The professional literature accentuates the need for mental health professionals to work towards building collaborative relationships with physicians. Mental health professionals are encouraged to prove their expertise through cases with successful outcomes, present credentials, learn the medical language, use brief and clear language while reporting back to physicians, and become a useful asset for physicians. Mental health professionals entering medical settings are advised that they will likely be faced with issues pertaining to hierarchical structures, and are encouraged to deal with these issues nonconfrontationally (Patterson, Peek, Heinrich, Bischoff, & Scherger, 2002). These authors propose that once the value of mental health professional's work is recognized, the issue of who is in charge tends to become less significant.

This present study addresses the limited overt attention to issues of power and particularly of gender in the medical family therapy literature. This current study arose from a qualitative study of the general experience of being a medical family therapist (Bischof, 1999). In the initial study, 13 medical family therapists practicing in nonacademic settings discussed their experiences, and issues of power and gender were quite evident, even though the study participants were not asked explicitly about these issues. This current investigation analyzed those initial transcripts for evidence of the influence of power and gender. Power was generally defined as having to do with one's place in the hierarchy, the ability to exert influence in decision-making, economic considerations, and how much accommodation was required to be included in the system. Gender issues included those explicitly identified as relating to one's gender or the gender of others in the system, as well as those reflecting socially constructed notions of feminine and masculine roles. After a discussion of the methods employed in this study, we offer a summary of the cases and a presentation of the major ways that gender and power were evident in their experiences. We conclude with some discussion of what was found and make suggestions for future consideration of power and gender issues in this growing area of medical family therapy.

METHOD

Research Design

This current study on power and gender issues in medical family therapy occurred as an outgrowth of an initial larger qualitative study by the first author (Bischof, 1999). Foci of the initial study included key opportunities and challenges of this work, how these therapists got involved in medical family therapy, and strategies they have found useful in collaborating effectively with health care providers.

The research design used in the initial study was a holistic, multiple-case, emergent design, and the individual family therapist was the unit of analysis. The exploratory nature of the study called for a flexible design that could be adapted to the emerging data (Goetz & LeCompte, 1984). The design utilized research methodology from the traditions of phenomenology, life history research, and survey research to explore the experience of being a family therapist in nonacademic medical settings. Nonacademic settings were targeted because the bulk of the literature up to that point had been published by and about medical family therapists in academic settings. Academic settings have by their nature a focus on education, and the "costs" of collaboration may be accepted as part of the educational mission. The initial study endeavored to explore medical family therapy in real-world clinical settings for these reasons. In-depth semi-structured interviews were conducted with all participants, and each completed a brief demographic and practice setting survey. The purpose of this current study was to identify specifically how issues of gender and power were manifested in the reported experiences of this group of medical family therapists.

Participants

Participants for the initial study were identified through several means. The first author reviewed the list compiled by the Working Group for Family Therapists in Medical Settings, and identified and contacted family therapists who were working in nonacademic medical settings, albeit a small number, as a large majority were involved in academic sites. Additional participants were identified through responses to posted announcements at relevant conferences or meetings (e.g., Family in Family Medicine Conference, Collaborative Family Health Care Coalition organizational meeting). Other participants were generated via snowball techniques from contacts with study participants and experts in the field. The first author also consulted with national leaders in the field of medical family therapy, especially later in the study, when attempting to identify participants who met specific criteria, such as those who were male, racial minorities, or those who worked in larger urban areas.

Several criteria were established to determine inclusion in the study. Some of the initial criteria were revised as the study progressed, to take into account the actual practice of medical family therapy as it emerged through early stages of the study. Presented here are the criteria that were used to arrive at the final sample for the initial study: (1) To ensure that participants held *family systems theory* as a primary theoretical perspective, a participant needed to be: (a) a graduate of a COAMFTE-accredited program, (b) a member of AAMFT or AFTA, (c) licensed/certified as a Marriage and Family Therapist, or (d) had significant family systems training and utilized this approach routinely in clinical practice (note: this final criterion was added to allow for the inclusion of more males in the study). (2) At least *two types of participants in terms of medical setting* were actively sought: (a) family therapists who were working in family medicine practices, and (b) family therapists who were working with other primary care specialties, such as obstetrics, internal medicine, or pediatrics, or other medical subspecialties. (3) To ensure that participants had *adequate experience* working in medical practice(s), a participant had experience working at least one day/week for at least one year. (4) An effort was made to ensure that the *gender and ethnicity* of participants reflected the gender and ethnic composition in the field.

As the study progressed, it became difficult to identify participants meeting some of these criteria, particularly to identify males or racial minorities who were doing this kind of work. In order to include more males, the criteria related to identification and training in family systems theory and therapy were expanded as noted above. Overall, there seemed to be a dearth of males doing collaboration in nonacademic medical settings. One prominent leader in the field remarked, "Boy, I can't think of anyone, what does that tell you?" Eventually, two males were included who did not meet the initial family systems experience criteria above (number 1, a-c above), but had been recommended by leaders in the field who were familiar with their work. One (case 11) had been a Clinical Member of AAMFT previously, and the other (case 12) had several years of clinical training and supervision in a family systems approach and held a systems orientation.

Leaders in the field from different geographic regions of the country who were contacted were unable to identify any racial minorities who were doing this work in nonacademic settings. According to one African-American man who worked in an inner city residency-based clinic with whom the first author spoke, it appeared that racial minorities in the field tended to be involved in inner city programs that typically included a residency training program or significant educational component. This did not fit with the purpose of the initial study, to access the experiences of those working in *nonacademic settings*. Thus, no racial minorities were included in the study.

The participants involved in this study collaborated with physicians from the following specialty and subspecialty areas: family medicine, internal medicine, pediatrics, obstetrics/gynecology, oncology, radiation oncology, neurology, reproductive endocrinology (infertility), rheumatology, and endocrinology.

A total of 13 participants were involved in this study. One participant (case 9) included in the study is a pediatrician/family therapist. He was included because his wife (case 8) is also a participant, they do co-therapy together, and he has had significant family therapy training. Summaries of the participants are included below.

Procedures

Potential study participants were contacted and screened based upon the above criteria. Those deemed appropriate gave their consent to participate and were asked to complete a brief demographic and experience/practice survey prior to being interviewed. Interviews were audiotaped and transcribed. Preliminary findings were mailed to study participants who were given the opportunity to make corrections or provide feedback before the final write-up.

In-Depth Interviews

In-depth, semi-structured interviews were conducted with the participants and served as the primary source of data in this study. All but two of the interviews were conducted face-to-face; the other two were done by phone. Interview length averaged approximately one hour, and ranged from 43 minutes to 80 minutes, with phone interviews tending to be slightly shorter.

Interview questions were open-ended and invited the participant to share his/her story. An attitude of partnership in the discovery process permeated the interviews. Participants were also asked to come up with a metaphor that encapsulated their experience working with health care providers in a medical setting. Probes were used throughout to clarify or elaborate upon responses (Patton, 1990). It should be noted that participants were not asked explicitly about power or gender issues in the initial study, but upon analysis for this current study, all revealed experiences that were related to power and/or gender.

Data Analysis

Initially, we will address some of the key elements of the data analysis from the initial study and then detail steps used in this current study. The first author employed data analysis strategies primarily from the tradition of phenomenological qualitative research (Boss, Dahl, & Kaplan, 1996; Moustakas, 1994; Polkinghorne, 1989) in the initial study.

These included several reviews and analyses of the transcripts and other sources of data (survey, field notes, documents obtained on site, contact summaries, and the first author's research journal reflections). To enhance the trustworthiness and dependability of the emerging findings, the initial study also employed the use of a 'devil's advocate' to question the development of emerging codes and themes. Further, participants were also provided a draft of the findings and were given the opportunity to correct or clarify the preliminary findings.

In order to understand the context of the initial larger study, the second and third authors read the entire dissertation report (Bischof, 1999). The first three authors then analyzed the complete transcripts of the interviews with focus upon identifying issues related to power and gender manifested in the interviews. Initial within-case analysis of the transcripts by the research team involved independent reading and coding to gather an overall sense of each participant and his/her experiences. Next, each transcript was carefully reviewed and coded independently by the researchers for incidence of issues relating to power and gender, utilizing constant comparison methods (Glaser & Strauss, 1967; Goetz & LeCompte, 1984). After this analysis, which included both within-case and cross-case analyses, the research team met to discuss their emerging findings and consensually developed a list of categories of issues addressed by the participants for both power and gender. This preliminary list was then taken back individually by each of the researchers to the transcripts for verification and modification. The research team met once again and consensually agreed upon a final categorization of the various experiences these medical family therapists reported related to power and gender in their work with health care providers in medical settings. These findings are presented below, following brief case summaries of the participants. These case summaries are included to provide some context and background for the voices of the participants in this study. We developed descriptive names for the participants to protect their anonymity. The names capture a significant theme or element of the participant's experience or practice. Names reflecting the actual gender of the participant have been used.

CASE SUMMARIES

Case 1: Medical Culture Molly, MS, RN, 41, is from the South. She is married to a physician and has a background in nursing, in which she saw a lack of attention to family and psychosocial issues. She shares space with an internist, and is the only therapist in a large multi-specialty medical facility, so she receives referrals from them and from other physicians in the community. She has an MS in MFT, specializing in Family Systems Medicine and possesses a keen sense of awareness of the culture of medicine.

Case 2: Entrepreneurial Jovial Judy, PhD, 52, is from the Midwest. She is married to a veterinarian. She practices in two separate facilities, one in a large metropolitan area, and the other in an outlying rural area. She enjoys her working relationships with the MDs, but has had difficulty with the office manager understanding the collaborative arrangement at one site.

Case 3: Relationship Rhonda, MSW, MA, 30, is from the Northeast. She is a certified sex therapist and began collaborative work in medical settings in a Human Sexuality Program in the Department of Family Medicine where she did her internship and then stayed on as staff for a while. For the two years prior to being interviewed she had worked in a family medicine group practice. She emphasized the importance of developing personal relationships with health care providers, something her departed predecessor at the group practice had not done very well.

Case 4: Rural Bowenian Jill, MS, 40, is from the Northeast. She is also a certified sex therapist and worked in the same Human Sexuality Program as did Rhonda above. For about 4 years she had co-taught an Introduction to Clinical Medicine course with a family physician. She employs a Bowenian family systems style of therapy and spoke about her goal of being a neutral presence in the medical settings she worked in, which were two rural practices. She was invited to collaborate in these rural practices as a solution to low job satisfaction of the MDs there.

Case 5: Managing Partner Rick, MA, MPA, 51, is from the Northeast. He had a previous career managing human service agencies and uses his managerial skills in his current rural collaborative practice. He is "unofficially" married to his family medicine collaborator. His medical setting is very integrated. He is also involved in a family systems medicine clinic in a Family Medicine Department.

Case 6: Radiation Onco-Consultant Barb, PhD, 35, is from the Northeast. She has a keen interest in mind-body connections. At the time of the interview, she had been involved for 4 years in the family systems medicine clinic for one day/week where she and Rick above supervise cases and conduct consultations. In the interview, she primarily focused on her work with a radiation oncologist, with whom she was consulting for five hours/week, offering him process-oriented feedback about his interactions with patients and staff.

Case 7: Visiting Onco-Jane, MS, 50, is from the Mid-Atlantic area. There is a strong tradition of nursing in her family of origin. She made a career change and left a tenured faculty position at a community college after her husband died of cancer. She was struck by the lack of attention to her and her husband's emotional needs as he suffered with cancer and she struggled in isolation as his primary caregiver. She works in a religiously affiliated nonprofit hospital system particularly with an oncologist, counseling cancer patients and their families, and terms her patient contacts as nonthreatening "visits."

Cases 8 and 9: Dr. & Mrs. Biopsychosocial, MD, 61, and MA, 59, respectively, are from a small town in the Upper Midwest. He is a pediatrician and the son of a family doctor who was one of the founders of the clinic where he now works. Having been exposed to MFT through his wife, and after two suicides in his practice, he was awarded a fellowship that gave him extended time off to pursue family therapy training. She has worked in a variety of mental health and hospital settings, and has collaborated with many physicians.

Case 10: Neophyte Nancy, MA, 43, is from a smaller town in the Midwest. She had always been healthy and had very little contact with physicians when an MD whom she knew through her church asked her to join a newly forming group of family physicians and provide mental health services on site there. With limited office space and another MD joining the practice, space was at a premium. Following a poorly communicated notice by the physician who had initially invited her to join the group, she left the on-site practice after a little over a year. She continued to receive referrals from the practice and stopped by regularly.

Case 11: Pragmatic Pediatrics Bob, PhD, 50, is from the Northeast. His primary professional affiliation is with Psychology, but he was a Clinical Member of AAMFT at one time. He is married to an ophthalmologist. He had been a reliable referral as a private practitioner for a group of pediatricians, and when they purchased the building, they invited him to join them at the pediatric practice on site for 1 1/2 days/week. Bob had extensive previous experience in medical settings, collaborating more than thirteen years with physicians. He came on board in part because of pragmatic reasons, and appreciated the convenience of being on-site.

Case 12: Mind-Body Michael, PhD, 41, is from a large metropolitan area in the Upper Midwest. His primary professional affiliation is with Psychology, but he had received extensive clinical training in marriage and family therapy. The son of a neurologist, he has a keen interest and considerable knowledge in health psychology and mind-body interactions. He worked at an HMO setting that has been held out as a model for collaborative health care for its highly integrated and sophisticated approach. He serves in an administrative role for collaborative care in the HMO, and has been involved in recent expansions of collaborative mental health services into subspecialty areas such as neurology, rheumatology, and endocrinology.

Case 13: Infertility Translator Martha, PhD, RN, 36, is from a large metropolitan area in the Midwest. Her mother was a nurse. Martha had worked for several years as a nurse in an infertility practice, and, as she learned about the field of MFT, went on to complete a PhD in the field. She performs a wide range of psychosocial services, including screening egg and sperm donors, grief counseling, and couples therapy. With her extensive medical background and sensitivity to the emotional impact of these problems and procedures, she often serves as a 'translator' for patients.

FINDINGS

The following two major sections comprise the primary findings of this study. We have divided issues of power and gender for organizational purposes, though it should be acknowledged that for some findings there is likely considerable overlap between power and gender, as these issues are often interwoven. This is especially true because the majority of participants were female and they were working mostly with male physicians and other health care providers and office staff who were female. Thus, what we report here in each section are issues that were explicitly identified as either related to power or gender, and other matters that seemed to involve principal attention to one issue or the other. In addition to reporting the findings in these areas, we intersperse some limited discussion as well.

Power Issues

Feminist family physician Lucy Candib (1995) describes traditional power in medicine as "power-over," or a kind of domination of one body over another. In the culture of medicine, the physician has traditionally held the position of power within the medical establishment. In this section we report significant areas related to power and hierarchy identified by the study participants. These issues regarding power fall into areas including the establishment of the collaborative relationship, accommodation, ongoing maintenance of the collaborative relationship, professional and practical considerations, and, finally, ways therapists seem to hold a one-up position at times.

Establishment of the Collaborative Relationship

In order for the therapist to get started doing this kind of therapy, several factors have to be considered. As the medical system is already more established, and considering that the therapist is the outsider entering it, the therapist is already in a one-down position of power from the start. Joining a medical system is akin to joining a family as one would do in therapy, and the best joining skills should be called forth. As Relationship Rhonda stated, "I think that I have found that I don't want to go in there with a bulldozer . . . doing it in a way, to help move them along, but not to be too threatening." She later emphasized the need to work on "building relationships" with the medical community. Her suggestions were echoed in the exhortations of Medical Culture Molly:

> One of the most important is to have a mutual respect for fellow therapists, and for the medical community, and not to go in there as "White Knight saviors" who are going to come in with this wonderful, magical stuff that we do that is non-pathologizing and non-medicinal. And if that's the attitude the therapist is going to have, the collaboration is going to be murder, absolute murder. We need physicians, physicians need us. . . . And never, never, never, never sermonize. Don't do it. Because the work that we do expresses what we do without having to sit there and give a speech about it.

Often medical family therapists have to 'sell' themselves and the benefits of their services to the physicians with whom they are considering collaborating. Therapists frequently need to justify their role in a medical setting. Several participants spoke about being in a position to convince physicians of the advantages of collaborating on-site, and even when some MDs were supportive, others in the setting seldom referred patients and seemed to devalue the role of the therapist. Managing Partner Rick described how he and his collaborating physician partner "sold ourselves as a unit to the board of directors of this non-profit corporation. In order to do what we wanted to do and also in order to have a hand in it, we said we'll do some of the management." In this particular case, not only did the therapist have to know family therapy, he also had to have the managerial background to be marketable to the medical system.

In some cases, therapists did free consultations in order to demonstrate how they might be of assistance. Managing Partner Rick stated his reason for doing so: "I don't want the economics to be another stumbling block in terms of getting me involved." It is less likely, of course, that a physician would offer free consults in order to get involved in a case.

In some cases, physicians and medical staff were not certain about the role the medical family therapist was to play. Others had some awareness of the potential role of a therapist on-site, yet operationalizing this role was a different matter. Therapists viewed their roles in various ways. While having primary responsibilities for treating patients for mental health and relational concerns, helping to reduce the burden on physicians and raising awareness about psychosocial issues were also important contributions. Rural Bowenian Jill reflected the multiple roles played by a medical family therapist:

> One of the things that was really stressed, that I tried to be sensitive to, coming from a Bowen Model, . . . when I was hired one of my concerns was coming into a system that was unfamiliar with a family therapist and wanting to come in and to be able to deal with that system as well as the patients. Also, if you feel like you have to come in as an equal to a doctor, you will never make it.

Medical family therapists often assumed they had to first seek to understand, and then be understood. Jill further stated, "So my goal was to come in and really be a neutral force and to work very slowly, understanding that if I went in and requested all kinds of things, I would alienate people, so I came in very low key."

Medical Culture Molly reiterated the need for the therapist to take responsibility in facilitating an effective entry into the culture of medicine:

> It just needs education on both sides, but if we're the ones that want to forge forward into collaborating with medicine, then we're the ones who need to get ourselves really well educated on what's going on in the medical world. . . . The only way we are going to be accepted–one of the only ways besides doing good work–is to understand their whole deal, just as any culture . . . we are the ones who have to understand their world to get accepted by them. And that's where I think many therapists fall short.

One of the male participants cautioned about assuming too much of a one-down position, and emphasized that therapists in medical settings need to claim their competence and recognize they have something valuable to offer. Mind-Body Michael advised:

> You bring a tremendously rich and informed and professional perspective to the health needs of the patient, and you can't go in with this sort of step-child attitude, or adoptive child attitude that they are the real authorities and we'll add our two cents if they allow us to. There's almost an institutionalized inferiority complex that I think you have to work to get over. . . . There are a number of things that re-emphasize that we are not necessarily looked at by the health system as of equal importance, but, damn it, don't come in there with the idea that you buy that! It tends to water down your effectiveness.

Accommodation Issues

A common theme revealed by participants in the study involved the need to accommodate to the culture of medicine and the needs of health care providers. Accommodation occurred in several different realms as articulated by study participants. These included accommodating to 'them' as in 'us versus them,' modifying one's style of therapy, and assuming that accommodation would not be reciprocated.

As the 'outsider' entering the culture of medicine, there may be significant ways therapists must adapt their styles in order to fit better with the pace of medical settings. Clinicians accustomed to having long conversations hypothesizing about the various contextual factors affecting a particular case learn to provide quick updates and concise summaries in their brief 'in the hallway' consultations with busy physicians. Mind-Body Michael likened the pace of medical settings to "the race between the tortoise and the hare. That they are running around from one to another very quickly, with a lot of confidence that in the end they will get to the finish line first." He saw his role as counter to this, patiently listening to patients' stories in order to gather an overall sense of what is going on. Medical Culture Molly warns that the family therapist ought to be cautious about debunking notions of individual psychopathology, "if you're going to be in someone's world, then you have to kind of go along with their languages. If I'm going to be with the physician and they're telling me that someone's depressed, and I say, oh, no, don't call them depressed, they're sad, I'm already going to distance that person." Study participants spoke to the need to be sensitive to and learn the language of the medical culture, consistent with previous medical family therapy literature.

Style of therapy. The approach to or style of therapy was another area in which therapists in this study noted a tendency to accommodate. Working in a medical setting in which an active orientation and time pressures are prevalent led some to alter their styles or begin to think differently about their own clinical work. Rural Bowenian Jill had been accustomed to seeing clients weekly for hour-long sessions, and with a family-of-origin therapeutic bent, tended to see clients over a longer period than proved optimal in her medical settings. A waiting list developed, as she was there only a limited number of hours per week, and was unable to see patients as quickly as the physician had hoped. This led her to adopt a briefer approach to treatment for some cases, and she had begun seeing people biweekly or for half-hour sessions to accommodate to the needs of the medical practice. Relationship Rhonda observed the following influences on her clinical work and the way she communicated about cases with physicians:

> ... the influence the physicians, or the medical setting has had on me. Which is–they have–part of their training, part of the way they go at things is to be very focused, very goal oriented, very treatment planning, and I think that's helped me be more tuned in, more on top of those things. . . . So, it's kind of helped me have a better focus–more direction. . . . Yes, it's definitely influenced my practice. I think just observing how they talk about cases, observing how they think about cases . . . even the questions that they would ask me. They're 'clean.' It's like they're very focused, precise . . . they would challenge me, too, to see how focused I am, if I was trying to explain what I was doing in therapy with a patient.

Other participants reported that working in a medical practice had led them to be more open to considering medications than family therapy colleagues in other settings, and were more inclined to inquire about medication side effects. Others asked more frequently about personal and family history of significant medical illness, even in their work in nonmedical settings, and some participants became more attuned to the family history of pregnancies and their effect especially upon female clients. Pragmatic Pediatrics Bob had some difficulty identifying exactly how working in medical settings had influenced his work, in part because of his extensive background in medicine, but he went on to reflect upon how the style he had developed is a nice fit with the culture of medicine and managed care as well:

> I have worked in so many medical settings. I know it completely shaped it, it just seems like part of the fabric. I'm very, 'what's the problem, what can we do to deal with it?' I am very comfortable with medicine. I think I am very kind of active, which is probably more also kind of a physician way to go about things. I want to 'fix the problem.'

Lack of reciprocity. Reflective of a power differential between medical family therapists and their medical collaborators, participants noted that accommodation was primarily unidirectional; there was a lack of reciprocity. Therapists did the bulk of adjusting to and adapting to the medical setting, and though they may have been frustrated by the lack of those in the medical culture accommodating to them, therapists typically did not expect that to occur. While some participants noted that over time they observed some subtle influences that their presence may have contributed to, this was viewed as a bonus, certainly not part of a balanced, reciprocal relationship. We conclude this section with strong words, perhaps revealing some ambivalence in his choice of language, from Managing Partner Rick as he poignantly sums up this tendency to accommodate and some of the potential payoffs for doing so:

> I try to accommodate myself to them, so I write in their charts and I use their lingo, and I learn their vocabulary, and I do the 15-minute consultations, and I do them for free. Maybe I am a whore, but I think that a combination of doing that for them gives me an entree that I don't find other therapists in the area that are just free standing therapists, even though they might be better than I am, have.

Maintenance of the Collaborative Relationship

Oftentimes, once the collaborative relationship was initiated, therapists had other issues in the collaborative relationship that they had to maneuver in order to continue working with the physicians. In certain cases, the physician would 'dump' his or her worst patients on the therapist as a way to deal with 'noncompliant' or with 'difficult' patients. Entrepreneurial Jovial Judy spoke about kidding her physician collaborator about these kinds of referrals, and that "sometimes he really doesn't want to deal with somebody, and they've become a hassle to him. He'll turn it over to us."

Another common occurrence is the physician unilaterally prescribing medication for a patient who was also being treated by the therapist, yet the MD did not consult with the therapist about beginning a course of medication. Neophyte Nancy shared some frustration with this, when "all of a sudden they are prescribing some kind of antidepressant without ever talking with me about it." Pragmatic Pediatrics Bob related a story about this as one of the more challenging aspects of his role as a therapist in a medical setting. Bob had been treating an adolescent and had considered the possibility of medication, yet had determined it would be prudent to wait and see if symptoms improved with continued therapy, only to find out at the next session that the MD had prescribed medication, without communicating with Bob about this. Bob explained from his experience that unsuccessful, poorly thought-out trials of medication provided a distraction from the therapeutic work. Bob debated about confronting the MD about this slight, yet he "wimped out" and failed to bring it up. Another participant directly confronted the physician about this practice, and the MD was agreeable, yet continued on in this unilateral decision-making regarding medication.

Confidentiality is another issue that medical family therapists have to deal with on a regular basis. Much about this topic has been addressed in the medical family therapy literature (McDaniel et al., 1992; Patterson et al., 2002; Seaburn et al., 1996). Issues typically revolve around expectations about sharing information, whether written releases are needed, how mental health services are documented, and differing values around public discussion of patient concerns and behaviors. Sometimes confidentiality was related to office space being shared with different staff having different job descriptions. Other study participants reported problems regarding charting and documentation. Mrs. Biopsychosocial expressed concerns about confidentiality, which was particularly germane for her in the small, rural community where she lived and worked: "Confidentiality and working here and again [my husband/colleague] is much more trusting of people. I have heard things that have gotten out that I am not at all happy about, and that is one reason I have reduced the number of notes I put down in the chart." Neophyte Nancy voiced other problems related to physicians' handling of confidentiality:

> They are not very good about confidentiality at all, and it seemed to me that they tended to think that they knew everything about a patient, but some patients don't tell them everything. They seem to

think that I should be willing to share anything I knew, too, and I was not willing to do that.

Professional and Practical Considerations

Some of the professional and practical considerations for the therapists included reimbursement issues, office space, interactions with office staff, and professional identity issues.

Reimbursement issues. In several cases, the MFT had difficulties with reimbursement issues that were never a problem for the physicians due to the nature of MDs' near universal reimbursement status in the health care system. Infertility Translator Martha reported "just problem after problem of reimbursement," while others termed these issues a "real struggle." In some cases the MFT was considered an employee of the physicians group, or would require the MD to sign off on their charts in order for therapy services to be reimbursable. One can see the inherent power issues in such financial arrangements and billing practices, with the therapist in some cases dependent upon the MD's status for professional and competent therapeutic services to be validated or approved. This issue was particularly relevant for some of the participants who worked in states that did not license MFTs. Such was the case for Rural Bowenian Jill, whose services were billed under the physician. She had some misgivings about her services being billed as if the MD were providing them, but that was the arrangement made by the health care system administrators, and permitted her to practice in that medical setting. Whereas, if she had to rely on billing under her credentials, she probably could not have practiced viably there. This, of course, raises ethical issues and places the therapist in a potentially vulnerable position. On the other hand, reimbursement constraints are often larger than the system of the practice itself. For example, some states require MDs to sign off on Medicaid treatment plans and reviews, placing both MFTs and MDs in uncomfortable situations.

Office space. Inadequate office space or lack of an office was another issue related to power dynamics that came up frequently. Visiting Onco-Jane had no real office to call her own. She described some of the challenges using medical exam rooms in the oncology practice where she met with patients to address their psychosocial needs. Sometimes therapeutic conversations had to be cut short "because somebody else needed to come in and use the space." Nurses and office staff learned to be sensitive to patients' needs, and try to allow for adequate time and privacy for emotionally distraught patients, yet, "if we are real busy, sometimes that can't happen and I can't get in the oncologist's way, so if he needs the room, he has first call on any room." Infertility Translator Martha expressed frustration with medical providers not understanding the benefit of having a consistent therapeutic space in which to conduct ongoing therapy, and that the MDs could not understand why she was "so upset that we've recommended you use whatever consult rooms that are available." Finally, Pragmatic Pediatrics Bob cited the windowless, dingy, basement office as the primary reason he opted to move out of his on-site practice. He had attempted to secure alternative office space in-house, but stated that the physicians seemed to have a much different sense of office space and did not seem to understand fully his concerns.

Interactions with office staff. Medical family therapy requires a high level of communication and negotiation skills that often will be tested by even the office staff in the medical setting. In one particular case, Entrepreneurial Jovial Judy mentioned that although the relationships with the physician group and the other mental health therapists were good, the relationship with the office manager often left much to be desired:

> . . . due to the office manager not understanding the concept of where we are coming from. She knows, because of our contractual arrangement that we make money for the doctor, so he likes us. But it's kinda sometimes hard to put us . . . and we often see ourselves in a one-down spot, as opposed to his practice. There's not as much care taken with our phone answering–getting dates, times, etc., whereas they wouldn't dare do that with him.

Professional identity issues. Visiting Onco-Jane stated the following about professional identity issues that MFTs may face in dealing with the medical community: "I think the primary struggle is just being recognized as a competent professional, someone who physicians feel comfortable referring patients to." Issues of professional identity were addressed by some of the participants as challenges related to their status. There was a lack of understanding about the role of a medical family therapist. Medical providers were more familiar with social work, which has had a longer tradition of working in medical settings. As the only AAMFT member in her local area, one participant claimed that medical professionals did not know what a marriage and family therapist was, "much less a medical family therapist." Issues of professional identity were especially prominent for those who had made a career change and struggled with finding their way as a novice in a new profession after having established themselves previously in some other career. Managing Partner Rick moved from directing large human service agencies to the "under belly" of the health care field as a family therapist. He saw himself as lower in the hierarchy than other more established mental health disciplines, such as social work and psychology, and complained of the "turf battles" that he encountered. A career change following the cancer-related death of her husband and struggles with professional identity were notably prominent for Visiting Onco-Jane, who was considering entering an MSW program to obtain a more recognizable and reimbursable degree:

> . . . it was a real challenge to switch careers at this point in my life. I felt that I was a very competent teacher. I loved teaching and I know I could have stayed there forever and been perfectly happy and I really did, I really loved teaching. So, learning to be a therapist and then deciding that I wanted to become a medical family therapist and now having to learn about illnesses and diseases and conditions that I didn't know about. And always kind of in the back of my mind, I am evaluating myself and comparing myself to the good, good teacher that I was. And then the learning therapist . . .

Medical Family Therapist in One-Up Position

Although the overwhelming considerations related to power for medical family therapists involve being in a one-down, less powerful position, some participants discussed how they were perceived as a threat to their medical colleagues, while others spoke to the influence they seemed to exert on the medical setting.

Being perceived as a threatening presence. Some participants believed that they were perceived as a threat to physicians simply by virtue of their being different and having a somewhat different style of relating. One speculated that some physicians are hesitant to collaborate with mental health professionals out of fear that they will be required to "look at their own stuff." A few had the sense that physicians were 'afraid' of them, and consequently shied away from the therapist. In the following two quotes, Radiation Onco-Consultant Barb speaks to this dynamic and then Neophyte Nancy describes her early experience with her physician group, and how things seemed to change when she was no longer on-site:

> Every once in a while there's this volleying around about my position and my relationship to him and him trying to figure it out. Is it

threatening or is it not threatening? It's really kind of fun to watch it play itself out.

At first they just avoided me like the plague and it's funny now that I'm gone [off-site], and I go back there, I think I'm less of a threat. I would get questions like, "are you psychoanalyzing me?" Which was intended as a joke . . . but I think they really wondered. I'd always kinda joke back. "Well, not unless you're going to pay me," and that kind of stuff . . . I think that just my presence kind of pushed them a little. I don't think that really pushed them real hard, but probably just in the sense that I tended to be more personable than they were used to being, but they experienced it as a push. I did have some of them make comments to me periodically, "you are different than anybody else I've ever met," things like that. . . . So, I think that just part of my presence and the way I have of thinking and talking about myself wasn't something they were used to.

Influencing mental health of medical setting. Another way that the medical family therapists seemed to influence the medical setting and the health care providers with whom they collaborated was through enhancing the overall mental health and well-being of the medical providers. This dynamic was mentioned by several participants. One noted that the therapist in a medical setting could help the physicians to "take better care of themselves." Another noted that often-serious and intense physicians tended to "lighten up" during interactions with her, due to her own easy style and sense of humor. This participant further remarked that once therapists get to know and respect the culture of medicine, health care providers will in turn, simply due to regular contact, "get educated in ours [the culture of family systems therapy] . . . they will have no choice." Relationship Rhonda connected her presence in the lives of those with whom she worked in the medical setting to some personal changes several of them made:

It's been interesting to just be a therapist in the office. I have noticed within the two year span people making shifts in terms of them personally . . . a few of them have asked me, "can I see you for therapy?" I've clearly said no, that's not a good idea, so I'm supportive and I give referrals a lot. But what I don't know, if people would have had the same openness to it–I think getting to know me and being exposed every week, you know, actually twice a week. I think that helps their openness. Some people have made some pretty major changes in their lives that I have observed in the last two years. . . . People got divorced, people got to therapy, people, you know got their husband to go to therapy and things got better. It's been very interesting . . . . Maybe it would have happened anyway, who knows, but I certainly have that curiosity. Particularly because they really came to talk with me, or . . . asked if they could come see me [for therapy].

GENDER ISSUES

Culture of Medicine–"Male"; Culture of Family Therapy–"Female"

The medical culture tends to be characterized as pragmatic, outcome-focused, action-oriented, and instrumental. The family therapy culture, in contrast, tends to be characterized as process-oriented in nature, emotionally expressive, abstract, and relationship-focused. The culture of medicine leaves little room for emotional expressiveness and displays of vulnerability, which are very often associated with a feminine style, and incompatible with a physician's typical role (McDaniel & Naumburg, 1988). These characterizations were also mirrored in the voices of the participants. Medical Culture Molly stated, "A lot of the physicians are more comfortable with machines." Pragmatic Pediatrics Bob commented, "I think I am very kind of active, which is probably more also kind of physician way to go about things. I want to fix the problem." In contrast, Entrepreneurial Jovial Judy had a slightly different experience with her physician collaborator who had previous training in social work:

> The other thing in collaborating, especially when I started my practice with him, he was really helpful on how to set up my own structure. He likes to sit and talk about that. That's probably from his background in the helping/counseling field, too. . . . He also challenges me at times to watch the number of hours I am working, like when he sees me there late at night.

Three other unique reflections came from participants surrounding the theme of a 'male' medical culture and a 'female' therapy culture. In commenting on her previous experiences as a patient and nurse, Medical Culture Molly stated boldly, "I hate male doctors," and saw it as part of her mission to address gender insensitivities:

As a patient I noticed a lot of demeaning attitudes toward females, and that bothered me a lot. And for many years I spoke and continue to speak to physicians about becoming more gender sensitized.

Interestingly, Molly showed a keen appreciation for the influence of the culture of medicine, and suggested that newcomers to medical settings view their role initially as similar to that of a cultural anthropologist. She was quite savvy in her regular communications with physicians, and was married to a physician, making her strong position on male doctors even more telling. She also described a very open, collaborative relationship she had developed with a female rheumatologist during some of her training that provided a welcome contrast to the male physicians she had typically encountered.

Neophyte Nancy, though, observed that the tendency for physicians to act and think in more stereotypical 'male' ways transcended the physician's gender:

The female doctor [of the five MDs in the practice] was also the Chief of Staff at the hospital. So she was only there part-time . . . less than the rest of them. But she thought very much like they [the male physicians] did. It was kind of weird.

Such experiences with female physicians may speak to the typical training of MDs in general, with an emphasis upon separate and procedural knowing, whereby staying separate and objective is preferred (Candib, 1995). Female physicians may experience a particular struggle between these preferred ways of knowing and their general socialization as women in which connected knowing in relationship is emphasized.

Mind-Body Michael, through his professional actions, seemed to be aware of these traditional gendered themes in medicine and made a conscious effort to address issues of gender in his setting. He explained his commitment to the importance of patients receiving services that showed sensitivity to diversity, including gender. In his highly integrated HMO setting, administrators typically placed mental health professionals in various medical practices in mixed-gender teams of two clinicians in order to promote gender sensitivity and to allow for increased collegial support.

Interestingly, three of the four males in this study were married to either a physician or their medical family therapy collaborator. Managing Partner Rick is a medical family therapist collaborating with his partner, a physician. Pragmatic Pediatrics Bob is a medical family therapist married to an ophthalmologist. Also, Dr. Biopsychosocial is in a collaborative relationship with his wife, Mrs. Biopsychosocial, a medical family therapist. A similar tendency seemed to be evident among the females in the study, that of being married to physicians or veterinarians. Three of the nine women, Medical Culture Molly, Entrepreneurial Jovial Judy, and Mrs. Biopsychosocial each shared this as their marital status.

Unique Role of Female Sex Therapists

Relationship Rhonda and Rural Bowenian Jill, along with being medical family therapists, are also certified sex therapists. This certification and expertise seemed to result in a slightly different relationship with physicians compared to the participants without this certification. These participants reported more positive interactions with physicians compared to the other, nonsex therapist participants. Physicians were reported to have called on these sex therapists for their expertise. One might make the assumption that there was a clear benefit for physicians having not just a medical family therapist available, but a medical family therapist with expertise in sexuality and sex therapy. Physicians are often minimally trained in human sexuality and may find it uncomfortable to address issues of sexuality with patients.

Rural Bowenian Jill related an experience that illustrates well the role that a medical family therapist with sex therapy expertise can play. Jill's male physician collaborator was conducting a routine physical exam with an adolescent male. During the exam the adolescent ejaculated unexpectedly. The physician immediately left the room, without saying anything to the patient, and contacted Jill. "Being a sex therapist I guess he also felt freer to call and ask me that question." She coached him on how to explain and normalize to this adolescent male what had happened, and bolstered the physician's confidence in being able to handle the awkward situation in a sensitive and professional manner. This situation is a good example of how physicians are able to use the expertise of medical family therapists, and in this case a certified sex therapist, for their own needs and the needs of their patients. Some of the participants with a background in nursing also seemed to benefit from their prior experiences with medicine.

The collaborative dyad of a female sex therapist and a male physician offers an intriguing gender-influenced relationship that challenges the stereotypical societal notion of the male possessing superior sexual knowledge and experience. The experiences of Jill and Rhonda suggest the possibility that female sex therapists can be intimidating to a male physician, especially a male physician without considerable expertise in sexuality. Yet, again, there seems to be some added respect for the therapist's expertise in this area. Rhonda commented about the first setting she worked in as medical family therapist and the uneasiness present between her and her physician collaborators. "I think it had to do with the discomfort of having therapists there. And I think that probably . . . not only are they therapists, they are sex therapists."

Gender Influences on Career

Several of the participants shared family of origin influences on their career choices and many of these were gender specific. These include career gender modeling, divergence in career paths related to gender, and family of procreation influences. Dr. Biopsychosocial explained that his father, a family physician for 47 years, influenced his decision to become a doctor, and Mind-Body Michael is the son of a neurologist. Although Mind-Body Michael did not choose a career in medicine, his therapy practice in health psychology keenly integrates mind-body connections, similar to his father's medical specialty.

Interestingly, some female participants had entertained the possibility of a career in medicine but ended up choosing a different path. Entrepreneurial Jovial Judy's family of origin and family of procreation were surrounded by medicine:

> I grew up with doctors. My great-grandfather was a doctor and we have lots of friends that are doctors. My husband is a veterinarian, which is a spin-off to the field, but the same kind of drugs, medicine.

Visiting Onco-Jane shared the history of female nurses in her family and the parallel history of male doctors in her family:

> My mother was a nurse. My aunt was a nurse. Two of my uncles were doctors, my former brother-in-law is a doctor, my sister is a nurse and my former sister-in-law is a nurse. I know I would have liked to have been a doctor. But I grew up in a time when women were more proscribed to go into nursing education, that kind of thing. So I became a teacher instead.

Infertility Translator Martha related a similar story about both her mother and grandmother being nurses. She also explained the diversity in her career path related to gender roles and expectations. Her path eventually led her to a doctorate in MFT.

> I met my husband, and decided I didn't want to work outside the home, so I went traditional, and switched from engineering to nursing, and ditched the notion of med. school. Then the smart part of me that was always told, you are too smart to be a nurse, then having gotten my master's and I was going to be a nurse practitioner.

Other participants like Relationship Rhonda, shared health and illness family of origin experiences that perhaps served as stepping stones to their chosen careers in the mental health professions. In Rhonda's family of origin, her father struggled from migraine headaches, her mother's health was compromised by obesity and her brother also struggled with cancer. In reflection, Relationship Rhonda believes these relationships and the role she played in her family probably shaped her role as a caregiver, and heightened her sensitivity to the influence of health issues on relationships.

Female–Educator Role; Male–Director Role

Three of the four male participants had either a director or management role in combination with their clinical roles. Managing Partner Rick attributed his managerial role to his management experience and interest. He shared that this role provided him with advantages such as being able to influence scheduling and enhancing his relationships with the nurses. He is clear that this managing role allowed him clout with the collaborating physicians and office practice. Dr. Biopsychosocial is the director of medical education in his large practice, along with his responsibilities as a pediatrician and part-time medical family therapist. Mind-Body Michael, too, is in a managing role. He manages the training for the large group of practitioners and is also the manager of the health psychology group itself. Interestingly, Mind-Body Michael mentioned several mentors in the interview; all were males in director or managerial positions.

Conversely, none of the female participants reported being in director or managerial roles, although both Rural Bowenian Jill and Relationship Rhonda assume educator roles. Interestingly, as noted above, these two participants are also certified sex therapists, and this expertise may lend it itself to an educational role. Infertility Translator Martha had significant responsibilities for patient education also. Medical Culture Molly also provides clinical supervision to interns practicing in medical settings.

This tendency for male medical family therapists to assume managerial or administrative roles in addition to their clinical ones may speak to the need for males in medical settings to have some status by position. This might contribute to their sense of authority or power, and counter the frequent 'one-down' position they may find themselves in as a therapist in a medical practice. Women may not have as much of a need to have a managerial position, but instead seem to rely for their satisfaction on their clinical skills and expertise, expressed through providing therapeutic and educational services. This finding may also be related to general patterns of patriarchy in medical and other systems in which men earn more money and are promoted to leadership positions faster.

DISCUSSION AND RECOMMENDATIONS

The previous sections included limited discussion about what some of these findings mean for family therapists who are or who are considering working in medical settings. Here we highlight some of the key points from this study, relate them to existing literature, and offer suggestions for further consideration of power and gender issues in medical family therapy. Given the nonrandom sampling and small sample size of this study, one should be cautioned about generalizing the findings presented to all medical family therapists in nonacademic settings. Conversely, as a qualitative phenomenological investigation, this exploratory study sought rich description of the pertinent experiences of therapists in medical sites, and was strengthened by including participants from diverse geographical regions who worked with a wide array of medical specialty areas.

This current study gleaned information related to power and gender from general discussions of the experience of being a medical family therapist. Though study participants were not asked specifically about power or gender, upon investigation, these influences were quite apparent. It would be interesting to speculate as to how the findings from this study would have been different if participants were asked directly about these issues. Although power has begun to be explicitly addressed in medical family therapy literature, overt attention to gender continues to be absent. Considering the findings presented here, future studies could more directly examine the dynamics related to power and gender for therapists in medical settings.

Earlier in the literature review, we discussed a model of five levels of collaborative care (Doherty, 1995; Doherty et al., 1996), each of which addressed issues of power in a different manner. Most of the participants in this study worked in settings that would be considered Level 3: Basic collaboration on site, while a few were in practices that were consistent with Level 4: Close collaboration in a partly integrated system. At these levels, respectively, the mental health professionals may resent the power imbalances, or view them as unresolved but manageable. These seem consistent with the experiences of the medical family therapists in this study. At the most integrated level there is a self-conscious effort to attend to team process issues and to balance power and influence among the collaborating professionals. The explicit attention to power and gender issues provided through this study may help to further discourse about these concerns in collaborative care. Continued efforts in this realm could also aid in making more fully integrated collaborative settings, complete with overt and sensitive consideration of issues of power and gender, a reality.

The current realities, though, described by study participants suggest that therapists working in medical settings should establish realistic expectations about their role in the system. Expecting to have an equal say in a balanced team simply sets one up for frustration and disappointment. Medical family therapists walk the fine line between assuming a secondary, yet important role. According to study participants, a therapist in a medical setting must both claim one's competence while recognizing the hierarchy inherent in the medical culture.

Power in the medical system was described earlier as 'power-over,' or male dominance in the physician-patient relationship (Candib, 1995). Candib offers an alternative conceptualization of power as 'power-to-empower,' drawn from a feminist perspective, in which power or influence is used to "empower the less powerful" (p. 244). She describes the benefits of connecting with patients in a meaningful, empathic way, in which they feel included and valued. Family therapists are in a position to empower patients by attending to them as whole people, taking into consideration their psychosocial and relational concerns, which may not be given much attention in systems that privilege the biomedical. Therapists in this study also described helping to empower health care colleagues to be more attuned to their own mental health and relational needs. Thus, while the prominent considerations related to power in medical settings focus on 'power-over,' a broadened perspective to include 'power-to-empower' may prove useful for medical family therapists trying to find their niche in the culture of medicine.

We noted earlier the lack of explicit attention to gender, particularly as it relates to the collaborative relationship. In a thought-provoking article by a family therapist and a family physician (McDaniel & Naumburg, 1988), the authors characterize gender as a 'family secret' in family medicine, the primary care medical field that has fostered much of early collaboration with family therapists. It seems that gender has also been a 'family secret' in the area of medical family therapy. McDaniel and Naumburg encourage better modeling of gender-sensitive attitudes, open discussion of gender issues, initiation of more flexible jobs to allow for a more balanced personal-professional life, and the extension of research that integrates a feminist perspective in the discipline of family medicine. These recommendations are relevant for medical family therapy, too. Indeed, this current study may help to advance dialogue about the role of gender in collaborative health care relationships.

Gender was also an issue in identifying participants for this study, and despite considerable efforts, it proved very difficult to identify males doing medical family therapy in nonacademic medical settings. This may be reflective of trends in mental health in general for females to hold master's level clinical positions, while PhD academics are more frequently males, where faculty positions or teaching roles add to their status. It may also be that the one-down nature of collaboration in medical settings proves to be a poorer fit for some males, who may have more difficulty tolerating this kind of relationship. The lack of identifiable males may also be related to the more masculine and instrumental nature of traditional western medicine. A female mental health professional may provide a more appreciable balance to the prevailing stereotypically masculine tendencies. Those in medicine, and perhaps even patients, may view these roles as more naturally suited to a female clinician. These possible explanations, along with consideration of the lack of racial minorities doing medical family therapy in nonacademic settings, deserve further attention in the future.

This study reveals gender-informed roles in the practice of medical family therapy. Male therapists tended to adopt managerial roles in addition to their clinical work, while females more commonly assumed educator responsibilities. Such roles may be important to consider for those contemplating work in medical settings, and flexible roles, not constrained by gender stereotypes, for both male and female medical family therapists should be encouraged.

Special expertise in sex therapy seemed to positively affect the work and status of two female therapists in particular. Many family therapists working in medical settings, especially those in subspecialty care, develop unique knowledge and expertise, and must learn about conditions, medications, and procedures specific to that specialty. Possessing special expertise may serve the family therapist, who is often trained as a generalist, in being viewed as more beneficial to one's medical collaborators. Competence in sex therapy seems to be helpful in the primary care setting, and medical family therapists would do well to gain capabilities in this or other specialized areas relevant to their medical settings.

A large number of medical family therapists in this study had physician spouses. Some of these couples practiced together in the same setting. Others conducted their professional work in separate contexts. These 'biopsychosocial' or 'medical-mental health' marriages have not been explored in the literature. It would be interesting to consider how these partners, with different professional backgrounds, influence one another through their intimate relationship. Indeed, Dr. Biopsychosocial reported that he had become more sensitive to gender issues in his medical practice because of his collaborative work with his wife. How is the professional work and personal life of each affected by their intimate relationship? How do these partners decide whether to work together professionally? How do power and gender play out in these marriages? The glimpses of biopsychosocial relationships from this study suggest that these unique unions warrant future examination.

Educating both the medical community and the mental health community on the value of collaboration and what each part brings to the partnership is vital to decreasing unbalanced issues of gender and power. A healthier environment can be created for both those providing care in the environment–therapists, physicians, and other health care providers, and for those receiving care–clients/patients, and their family members. As the professionals progress in their ability to directly discuss how issues of power and gender are at play in their working relationships, it is likely that these issues will be more conscious as well in interactions with clients/patients and family members. Modeling a healthy balance of gender and equality in the partnerships between physicians and therapists may be mirrored also in the care provided to those they serve. "The energy that flows between people when this partnership occurs can carry the work through the inevitable adversity and challenges, and sustain their vision of [what is possible in] health care" (Patterson et al., 2002, p. 170).

REFERENCES

Bernard, C. B. (1992). Counseling psychologists in general hospital settings: The continued quest for balance and challenge. *The Counseling Psychologist, 20*(1), 74-81.

Bischof, G. H. (1999). Medical family therapists working in non-academic medical settings: A phenomenological study (Doctoral dissertation, Purdue University, 1999). *Dissertation Abstracts International, 60,* 5428.

Boss, P., Dahl, C., & Kaplan, L. (1996). The use of phenomenology for family therapy research: The search for meaning. In D. H. Sprenkle & S. M. Moon (Eds.), *Research methods in family therapy* (pp. 83-106). New York: Guilford.

Campbell-Heider, N., & Pollock, D. (1987). Barriers to physician-nurse collegiality: An anthropological perspective. *Social Science Medicine, 25*(5), 421-425.

Candib, L. M. (1995). *Medicine and the family: A feminist perspective.* New York: Basic Books.

Doherty, W. J. (1995). The why's and levels of collaborative family health care. *Family Systems Medicine, 13,* 275-281.

Doherty, W. J., McDaniel, S. H., & Baird, M. A. (1996). Five levels of primary care/behavioral healthcare collaboration. *Behavioral Healthcare Tomorrow, 5,* 25-27.

Glaser, B. G., & Strauss, A. L. (1967). *The discovery of grounded theory: Strategies of qualitative research.* New York: Aldine.

Goetz, J. P., & LeCompte, M. D. (1984). *Ethnography and qualitative design in educational research.* San Diego: Academic Press.

Good, G. E. (1992). Counseling psychologists in hospital/medical settings: Dilemmas facing new professionals. *The Counseling Psychologist, 20*(1), 67-73.

McDaniel, S., Hepworth, J., & Doherty, W. (1992). *Medical family therapy: A biopsychosocial approach to families with health problems.* New York: Basic Books.

McDaniel, S. H., & Naumburg, E. H. (1988). Gender issues: Family medicine's family secret. *Family Medicine, 20*(6), 408-410.

Moustakas, C. (1994). *Phenomenological research methods.* Thousand Oaks, CA: Sage.

Patterson, J., Peek, C. J., Heinrich, R. L., Bischoff, R. J., & Scherger, J. (2002). *Mental health professionals in medical settings: A primer.* New York: Norton.

Patton, M. Q. (1990). *Qualitative evaluation and research methods,* (2nd ed.). Newbury Park, CA: Sage.

Polkinghorne, D. E. (1989). Phenomenological research methods. In R. S. Valle & S. Halling (Eds.), *Existential-phenomenological perspectives in psychology.* New York: Plenum.

Seaburn, D., Lorenz, A., Gunn, W., Gawinski, B., & Mauksch, L. (1996). *Models of collaboration: A guide for mental health professionals working with health care practitioners.* New York: Basic Books.

Shields, C. G., Wynne, L. C., McDaniel, S. H., & Gawinski, B. A. (1994). The marginalization of family therapy: A historical and continuing problem. *Journal of Marital and Family Therapy, 20,* 117-138.

Sweet, S. J., & Norman, I. J. (1995). The nurse-doctor relationship: A selective literature review. *Journal of Advanced Nursing, 22*(1), 165-170.

Popcorn Moments:
Feminist Principles
in Family Medicine Education

Mary E. Dankoski
Shobha Pais
Kathleen A. Zoppi
Jennifer S. Kramer

SUMMARY. Feminist principles are rare in medical education and in the practice of medicine. The authors are feminist family therapists and feminist health communication scholars who are faculty in a department of family medicine. In this paper, they present their use of a feminist perspective and feminist methods in their teaching of family physicians in training. The use of a live supervision practicum, imported from marriage and family therapy training, is described as an example of how

Mary E. Dankoski, PhD, is Assistant Clinical Professor, Department of Family Medicine, Indiana University.

Shobha Pais, PhD, is Adjunct Assistant Clinical Professor and Behavioral Science Director, Department of Family Medicine, Indiana University.

Kathleen A. Zoppi, PhD, MPH, is Associate Clinical Professor, and Director of Fellowships and Faculty Development, Department of Family Medicine, Indiana University.

Jennifer S. Kramer, MS, is a doctoral candidate, Department of Communication, Purdue University.

Address correspondence to: Mary E. Dankoski, Indiana University, Department of Family Medicine, Family Practice Residency, Indianapolis, IN 46202 (E-mail: mdankosk@iupui.edu).

[Haworth co-indexing entry note]: "Popcorn Moments: Feminist Principles in Family Medicine Education." Dankoski, Mary E. et al. Co-published simultaneously in *Journal of Feminist Family Therapy* (The Haworth Press, Inc.) Vol. 15, No. 2/3, 2003, pp. 55-73; and: *Feminist Perspectives in Medical Family Therapy* (ed: Anne M. Prouty Lyness) The Haworth Press, Inc., 2003, pp. 55-73. Single or multiple copies of this article are available for a fee from The Haworth Document Delivery Service [1-800-HAWORTH, 9:00 a.m. - 5:00 p.m. (EST). E-mail address: docdelivery@haworthpress.com].

http://www.haworthpress.com/web/JFFT
Digital Object Identifier: 10.1300/J086v15n02_03

feminist family therapists can bring a much-needed but rarely taught perspective to medical education. This perspective represents a paradigm shift away from the traditional model in medicine, one that is based on objectivity and separateness, to a more empathic and connected stance which shifts power in the physician-patient relationship. *[Article copies available for a fee from The Haworth Document Delivery Service: 1-800-HAWORTH. E-mail address: <docdelivery@haworthpress.com> Website: <http://www.HaworthPress.com> © 2003 by The Haworth Press, Inc. All rights reserved.]*

KEYWORDS. Medical family therapy, marriage and family therapy, feminist family therapy, feminism, family medicine, medical education, doctor-patient relationship, health communication, feminist pedagogy

INTRODUCTION

Medical family therapy offers marriage and family therapists (MFTs) many new clinical practice and research opportunities. In addition to clinical practice, however, MFTs can bring unique skills and perspectives to medical education. Feminist family therapists, in particular, bring content, methods, and conceptualizations to medicine that are generally lacking during most physicians' medical school and residency training. The authors are faculty in a family medicine department, trained as feminist family therapists (MED and SP) and feminist health communication scholars (KAZ and JSK). We draw on our use of a live supervision practicum–a common training experience in MFT programs, but rare in medical education–as an example of how we use feminist family therapy process in our teaching of family practice resident-physicians. The feminist content and processes we use in our teaching and supervision represent a shift from the traditional medical model of knowing to a more connected knowing. This is not only a paradigm shift for the physician, but a shift of power dynamics in the doctor-patient relationship into a more collaborative and relationship-centered stance.

We briefly will review feminism in marriage and family therapy and medical education, live supervision in family therapy and in family medicine, then will discuss the specific feminist processes we use through the practicum training experience to encourage such a power shift. A case example will also be presented.

Feminism and Marriage and Family Therapy

Feminists have been instrumental in calling attention to issues of power and responsibility in relationships, and to therapists taking active stands in the therapeutic process (e.g., Avis, 1992; Bograd, 1992; Kaschak, 2001; Mirkin, 1990; 1994; Wright & Fish, 1997). The earliest feminist critiques of family therapy raised the awareness of implicit sexism in many family therapy theories that maintained a view of the two-parent, heterosexual, patriarchal family as the norm (Luepnitz, 1988; Walters, Carter, Papp, & Silverstein, 1988). Additionally, early critiques centered on problems inherent in the neutrality maintained by traditional systems thinking which implied that, despite power differences, all members of a family were equally responsible for their interactions (see Ault-Riche, 1986; Braverman, 1988; Goldner, 1985; Goodrich, Rampage, Ellman, & Halstead, 1988; Hare-Mustin, 1978; Taggart, 1985). More recent feminist literature has addressed multiple social indicators such as ethnicity, sexual orientation, and socioeconomic status in addition to gender (e.g., Bryan, 2001; Hines, Garcia Preto, McGoldrick, Almeida, & Weltman, 1999; Johnson & Colucci, 1999; Kliman & Madsen, 1999; McGoldrick, 1998; Prouty & Bermudez, 1999), as well as critiquing research methods (e.g., Avis & Turner, 1996; Dankoski, 2000), and training and supervision theories and processes (see Ault-Riche, 1987; Crespi, 1995; Prouty, 2001; Prouty, Thomas, Johnson, & Long, 2001; Wheeler, Avis, Miller, & Chaney, 1985; Weingarten & Bograd, 1996). For example, a thorough statement of feminist supervision that has been influential in our work is the chapter by Porter and her colleagues (1997). These authors met as a working group to reflect and developed a comprehensive definition of feminist supervision that they called "covision." They articulated several principles that guide feminist supervision, including: proactively analyzing power between the supervisor/supervisee, the therapist/client, and within the client's relationships, the development of a mutually respectful, collaborative relationship with supervisees which also accounts for their developmental level; attending to context, diversity, and the role of language in social construction processes; facilitating and modeling self-examination and reflexivity as part of professional development; maintaining ethical standards; and advocating for social change. Feminist supervisors teach content that is consistent with feminism, and also use and model feminist processes in their teaching and supervisory relationships.

Live Supervision in Marriage and Family Therapy Training

A substantial part of marriage and family therapy clinical training is accomplished through live supervision, in which supervisors observe sessions as they are conducted, often through one-way mirrors or via closed-circuit video cameras, to provide learners with feedback in the immediate teaching moment. Montalvo and Storm (1997) summarize the benefits of live supervision to both supervisors and supervisees. They note that supervisors who promote live supervision believe that this method provides a supportive environment in which supervisees can learn a new skill. They also believe that this method creates opportunities for therapists to try out new behaviors in the moment, which thereby accelerates learning. Supervisors can help trainees who are stuck by suggesting alternatives that might not otherwise be considered by supervisees. Additionally, supervisors can gain critical information such as responses of supervisees, client reactions, or therapeutic interactions that may be overlooked or unintentionally ignored in other forms of supervision, such as case consultation. If there are other trainees observing the session, they can observe and learn without the pressure of being responsible for the encounter, with the luxury to assess and discuss alternate possibilities. In the context of live supervision, supervisors can supervise by selectively commenting on the session, requesting supervisees to pay attention to the session in a particular way, and/or asking for opinions to tap into their perspective and thinking. Proponents further believe that the supervision process generates multiple perspectives, which is a benefit to both therapists-in-training and to clients. We believed that these opportunities afforded by the live supervision process would benefit our residents and the patients of our family practice center.

Feminism and Medicine

Many feminist critiques of medicine arose in the 1970s during the time of that women's movement, and focused mainly on women's empowerment through learning about their bodies (Candib, 1995). Additionally, feminists raised the awareness of how women have been treated by the medical system, for example, by having their symptoms blamed on their reproductive systems (Candib, 1989), being over-medicated with tranquilizers (Albino, Tedesco, & Shenkle, 1990), and being excluded from clinical studies (Burge, 1991). This women's health movement was directed largely by self-help initiatives outside of medicine, and many women became mistrustful of physicians (Ruzek, 1978). During this same time period, more women became physicians, yet powerful socialization forces existed that often placed physicians in a bind of displaying qualities of traditionally socialized men in order to succeed (Hamilton, 1994; Walter, 1988). This pressure to exhibit instrumental characteristics traditionally associated with male socialization, such as competitiveness and rational intellectualization, limits both male and female physicians from being more intuitive, acting more relationally, or from being in touch with their emotions in clinical encounters. Within medicine, many physicians are reluctant to use the term "feminism" because it is perceived as divisive and reactionary. While many physicians have become more involved in advocating for the women's health movement, this is not necessarily the same as a feminist approach to medicine. However, a feminist critique from within medicine that has been highly influential in our work with family medicine residents was written by Lucy Candib, MD (1995), in which she examines what a feminist medical relationship might look like.

Candib (1995) argues that the contemporary construction of the doctor-patient relationship as a contract promotes a marketplace, consumerist approach to healthcare. The contractual approach, while advocating for patient choice, ignores the enormous power differences that exist between a doctor and patient and creates potentially adversarial relationships. Instead of viewing healthcare as a product to be bought and sold, she offers a feminist "being-in-relation" approach to clinical relationships. This stance places caring and trust at the heart of the doctor-patient relationship, in opposition to an emphasis on objectivity and rationality, and highlights the potential healing and nurturing that can occur within relationships of unequal power. While this is not new to feminist family therapists (see also Doherty & Campbell, 1988), it is a new and provocative paradigm challenge within clinical medicine.

One reason this paradigm shift is so provocative is that it goes against the way physicians are taught to think throughout their medical education. Much of medical education occurs at the levels of procedural knowing and separate knowing (Belenky, Clinchy, Goldberger, & Tarule, 1986). Procedural and separate ways of knowing are based on critical thinking, objectivity, and reason, and are a large part of the professional socialization into medicine (Candib, 1995). Knowing procedurally how to conduct clinical exams and remaining objective or separate from the patient are useful when learning about the science of medicine, assessing and diagnosing disease, and predicting prognosis based on scientific evidence. However, they are limited for learning about the person living the illness and may often be experienced as distant and sterile. Both of these ways of knowing actively exclude the self from the process, as opposed to the level of connected knowing, in which knowledge comes through personal experience, an understanding of context, and empathy (Belenky et al., 1986).

Connected learners are by no means less analytical or poor at critical thinking. They establish a holistic stance towards information and arrive at their conclusions via a different route. Methodologies which work best for connected knowers tend to be collaborative and, hence, interactive. We believe that physicians should be able to integrate multiple ways of knowing, and that the art of medicine lies in the ability to draw on connected knowing. This also opens up feminist avenues for healing, patient empowerment, and social change. Physicians can show this kind of feminist relational caring and empowerment in their clinical practices by expressing genuine feelings and empathy, attending to meaning and context, making a patient feel known, respecting him or her as a person, recognizing oppression, acknowledging choice and control, using a patient's language, and through patient education (Candib, 1995).

Live Supervision in Family Medicine Behavioral Science Training

While national medical school curriculum guidelines in the United States do include some behavioral science education for all medical students, much of it is content-focused rather than skill-focused, covering psychiatry topics, individual development, and some social issues, for example. Other than psychiatry rotations, opportunities are generally few for medical students to experience focused skill-development educational interventions in the behavioral science arenas. However, one of the things that makes post-graduate training in family medicine unique is that it is the only medical specialty that requires a nonphysician faculty to teach a structured curriculum in behavioral science. While other specialties, such as internal medicine, require some behavioral science curriculum, it is not necessarily required to be taught by a nonphysician, although it often is (Accreditation Council for Graduate Medical Education, 2003). A wide variety of disciplines teach behavioral science curriculum across family medicine programs, including MFTs, psychologists, social workers, and health communication experts. Content areas required in behavioral science curriculum include, among many: psychiatry topics (e.g., depression, anxiety), chemical dependency, family and individual development, cultural competency, communication skills, and counseling skills (Accreditation Council for Graduate Medical Education, 2001).

Some family practice residencies have used live supervision models in their training of family practice residents (e.g., Susan McDaniel, PhD, and her colleagues in Rochester, NY; see also Patterson, Bischoff, & McIntosh-Koontz, 1998; Patterson, Scherger, Bischoff, & McIntosh-

Koontz, 1998); however, it is more common in residency programs to teach counseling skills through didactic sessions and/or through counseling clinics and co-counseling sessions (where a behavioral science faculty and resident see a patient jointly; Johnson, 1999). Many programs also offer process-oriented education focused on doctor-patient relationship issues, such as Balint groups which are designed to process difficult patient interactions and physician personal emotional responses to their patients (Scheingold, 1988).

Thus, family physicians as a group receive far more education in the behavioral sciences and tend to be more integrative and interdisciplinary than other medical specialties. Indeed, the discipline of family medicine is based on the biopsychosocial model, first proposed by pioneering physician George Engel (1977; 1980). The biopsychosocial model acknowledges the interdependent relationships between the biological, psychological, individual, family, and community contexts of health and illness. Family therapists have enjoyed a long partnership with the discipline of family medicine, and have been instrumental in developing systemic, integrative training programs and models of patient care for both family physicians and family therapists (e.g., Doherty & Baird, 1983; 1987; Doherty, Baird, & Becker, 1987; McDaniel, Campbell, & Seaburn, 1990; McDaniel, Campbell, Wynne, & Weber, 1988; McDaniel, Hepworth, & Doherty, 1992; Patterson, Peek, Heinrich, Bischoff, & Scherger, 2002; Seaburn, Lorenz, Gunn, Gawinski, & Mauksch, 1996).

The work of these innovators provides a solid foundation for our clinical practices as MFTs and in our teaching of the behavioral science curriculum. Yet, because 70% of mental health problems are treated in primary care in this country (Fisher & Ransom, 1997) and because family physicians spend a great deal of time counseling patients on important health management issues, we have chosen to emphasize counseling skills training in our behavioral science curriculum. Like many other residencies, our initial attempt was to engage the residents in co-counseling experiences. The intent of the co-counseling learning experience was to allow residents to spend an hour with their own patient along with a behavioral science faculty present, during which the resident was expected to take the lead. However, the process often became one where the resident spent the hour with a patient seen by the MFT faculty for ongoing therapy, but who was not previously known to the resident. This typically resulted in the resident sitting silently while the MFT faculty and patient tried to bring the resident up to speed with the therapeutic process. This ended up being disjointed for the patient and a suboptimal learning experience for the resident. As a result, the practicum model from marriage and family therapy training was imported into the behavioral science training of family practice residents. This is a common model in MFT programs, yet is unusual and unique in medical education.

Because medical students have relatively few opportunities for focused training in counseling skills as discussed above, we considered it to be developmentally appropriate to use live supervision as the modality to teach these skills. Similar to the reactions of novice therapists to the live supervision process (Liddle, Davidson, & Barret, 1988), novice resident physician supervisees were initially worried about being judged as incompetent, and therefore were preoccupied with their performance and supervisory evaluation. It was important to make sure that supervisees did not view the process of live supervision as disempowering. Although critics of live supervision have stated that supervisees can become overly dependent on their supervisors, lack self-confidence, and/or become deskilled (Montalvo & Storm, 1997), we were not concerned this would happen since resident physicians had been seeing their patients independently for routine patient care visits in our family practice office for at least a year and a half of training before getting trained in counseling skills. Family practice residencies are three years in length; the practicum experience begins early in year two and spans about 18 months.

Teaching Therapy Skills Through a Live Supervision Practicum

Practicum begins as part of a two-week behavioral science block rotation during which residents receive intensive teaching in small groups on a variety of topics, including a didactic session on basic therapeutic skills and models of psychotherapy. For example, since residents are expected to spend about an hour with their patient in practicum–a luxury compared to a typical fifteen-minute office visit–they are provided with information about basic skills such as blocking, redirecting, reflection, and reframing, and are taught more advanced family therapy interventions based on the biopsychosocial model (see McDaniel et al., 1992). Over the next 18 months, residents are scheduled with three or four of their peers for a practicum afternoon approximately once every other month until they graduate. Each resident is asked to invite a patient of his or her choice and independently schedule the patient for an hour. As family therapists, we also emphasize the importance of inviting the patient's family whenever possible and appropriate.

The structure of our practicum sessions with residents is similar to the training of two of the behavioral science faculty in MFT (MED and SP). In a 15-minute pre-session, the resident is invited to describe the patient, his or her family, and the goals of the session. The group of residents and behavioral science faculty observe the session in the precepting room through a closed-circuit television monitor, and often engage in dialogue with each other about the process of the session as the session is taking place. The resident conducting the session takes a mid-session break, the goal of which is twofold. First, it provides an opportunity for the resident to receive feedback from the faculty and process their thoughts about the session and personal reactions to the patient. Second, it gives an opportunity for the learner group to provide some feedback both to their colleague conducting the session and for the patient. After the session is completed, a 15-minute post-session is conducted with the entire group to process the session, identify skills learned and employed during the session, as well as co-construct a treatment plan that now includes both biomedical and psychosocial aspects of the patient's life.

Specific Feminist Processes Used in Practicum

In our work through the behavioral science curriculum and particularly in practicum, we teach feminist-informed content, use feminist processes in our teaching and supervision, maintain a feminist perspective in case discussions and interventions, and recognize the parallel processes between the physician-patient and the supervisor-supervisee. We also use the foundational principles of feminist supervision as outlined by Porter and her colleagues (1997), especially proactively analyzing power issues, developing collaborative and supportive relationships, attending to the developmental level of each resident, and modeling reflection and self-examination. Many of these are discussed in more detail below.

Collaboration. Throughout the practicum process, we make a conscious decision as educators not to direct the resident physicians to engage in any specific manner with their patient(s) or practice any specific skills during the practicum session. This nondirective, feminist, collaborative approach is contrary to the highly directive and problem-based model of medical training. The traditional medical model teaches one to examine, make a diagnosis, and decide what needs to be done with the problem. Instead, we expect the residents to listen attentively to their patient and not have to change or fix anything. The only direction the residents are typically given when asked is to 'just be' with their patients, learn about their lives, their perspective of their health condition, and elicit their expectations of the visit.

However, residents are also monitored in their ability to manage anxiety they experience during the session. It is not unusual for residents to come back to the precepting room during the mid-session break and be surprised at the psychosocial issues they have been informed about by the patient. Sometimes the residents are clearly overwhelmed with the information, which causes considerable anxiety as they believe they have to do something about it, and feel an incredible sense of responsibility for their patient's social and psychological well-being. Depending on the resident's developmental level and the type of issue (i.e., if there is a safety risk for the patient, such as interpersonal violence), we often provide clinical direction, in a collaborative and respectful way. But for the most part, we encourage them to stay with their anxiety, and to continue to 'be' with their patient as appropriate. This paradigm shift is so markedly different from the typical directive approach in medicine that residents often struggle. However, in this struggle beyond their comfort zone, most grow far more confident and relationally skilled in the psychosocial aspects of practicing medicine. Many are surprised to receive positive feedback from patients regarding the practicum visit, when they may personally feel they did not 'do' anything, yet in the patient's eyes they provided good medicine by listening and connecting with them.

Safety Within a Group Process. The process of learning therapy skills through the practicum is also nontraditional in medicine in that it allows the learners to participate in a cohort group. As residents spend time together throughout their behavioral science curriculum, they move from being a collection of individuals to becoming a cohesive group, which in many cases becomes an essential part of the learning process. As educators, our role is to promote a safe climate for collaborative learning, and to encourage and facilitate meaningful dialogue between the learners and the faculty. Often during the mid-session break, residents within a cohort group actively engage in critical reflection and are open to new ideas and perspectives from their colleagues and faculty. Each individual's feedback is also encouraged during the post-session. Additionally, the members in the cohort group often give each other moral support during the mid-session break and post-session, which creates connectedness among them. The group also nurtures individual success and learning. This group process differs markedly from how physicians-in-training are typically taught during their residency.

Self-Reflection. Besides the practicum as a place of safety and learning connected knowing, the behavioral science curriculum provides a multitude of opportunities for reflection and experiential learning. As part of the longitudinal curriculum, residents spend time during the two-week behavioral science rotation working on their own personal genograms. "Self-of-the-physician" issues are addressed in the context of patient care through discussions about caring for patients with whom they have struggled. There is also a monthly group that focuses on patients that residents consider "difficult" and their personal reactions to them. We attempt to know our residents as persons, understand their context, and show genuine emotion and empathy within our teaching relationships with them, parallel to what Candib (1995) recommends for a feminist physician-patient relationship. These opportunities are created specifically to allow residents to engage in a self-reflective learning process that is safe and empowering, a process not usually actively encouraged in medical education. All of these processes form an integral part of feminist pedagogy, which emphasizes collaborative and interactive learning by shifting the focus of attention from the teacher to the learners.

Empathy and Empathic Listening. We emphasize empathic listening throughout the behavioral science curriculum. Empathy is the capacity to understand and respond to the unique experiences of another, and empathic listening is always centered on the other person with the goal of making them feel uniquely understood (Jordan, 1991). Empathic listening is the highest expression of the art of listening (Ciamamicoli & Ketcham, 2000). As educators with a goal of teaching about the physician-patient relationship, it is our belief that empathy is a feminist issue and that an empathic relationship can provide healing opportunities. While many nonfeminist physicians practicing from a separate knower perspective maintain that empathy is important in clinical practice, it is often reduced to a technique (i.e., saying a certain phrase) or a means to an end, such as making a visit more efficient (Candib, 1995). This construction of empathy does not require a physician to actually care about the patient, and it allows the physician to remain separate. A connected knower's definition of empathy acknowledges the effects of empathic caring on the physician. A clinical practice based on empathy and being-in-relation recognizes that daily encounters with patients personally impact and transform the provider (Candib, 1995).

The difference between empathy/empathic listening and sympathy/sympathetic listening (which is a passive experience of sharing another person's emotion) is defined for residents. It is not surprising to observe residents shift their current opinion of their patients after the counseling session. The emotional aspects of the sessions often bring new insights and understanding about the lives of the patients and create a new dimension in the physician-patient relationship. During practicum sessions, we have observed several resident physicians who had initially expected to learn very little find that patients shared important and vulnerable stories about their lives. Residents often state that their relationship is stronger with their patient after a practicum session, and that they will provide care differently based on what they learned about their patient's story. This care is often less focused on purely biomedical issues and is less hierarchical. Rather, it is more collaborative, systemic, and relationally focused because of the resident's increased understanding of the patient's perspective.

Initial Challenges Introducing Practicum into the Curriculum

The practicum process has been in existence in our residency curriculum for three years, and the change from co-counseling to the counseling practicum was a challenge initially. This included requesting an additional six half-days of behavioral science curriculum time over an 18-month period, from a complex scheduling system in which curriculum time is highly protected because of the breadth of information that must be taught in family medicine. To gain the acceptance and support of our physician faculty colleagues, we needed to educate them about the importance and value of the model as well as the process of group learning, since it is foreign to their own training. More importantly, we had to educate the residents about practicum and the expectations we had for the process. Initially, many residents expressed discomfort and fear of being observed on camera, having to practice psychosocial skills for almost an hour, and raised questions about the utility and practicality of these sessions for their future clinical practices. However, we have observed that as they become familiar with our expectations, experience the supervision process as occurring within a spirit of support rather than criticism, develop safety within their cohort group, and experience changes in their relationships with their patients, this resistance lowers significantly. Over the years, residents have incorporated "practicum" into their vocabulary and some have even requested live supervision outside of the set, required schedule.

We provide a case example below to explain how many of the processes described above have been used in practicum sessions. The session was a turning point in the understanding and practice of a collaborative biopsychosocial clinical stance of the physician described.

CASE EXAMPLE

Dr. Smith (names in case example are changed to protect confidentiality), a 2nd year resident, is a single, white, Christian male in his mid-twenties who completed his medical education in the Midwestern United States. For his first practicum counseling session, he invited a female African American patient named Jeanette who was in her early 40s, who he had been treating for depression with antidepressant medication. Dr. Smith invited her because he had a 'gut-level' feeling that more was going on with her than he knew. During the pre-session, he stated that his goal for the session was to find out more about her current and past family history. He also had a hypothesis that she might be in a physically abusive relationship.

Dr. Smith began the session by asking about her family history, and the patient disclosed within the first 10 minutes that she had previously been in a physically and emotionally abusive marriage, was currently divorced, and was dating someone else. Dr. Smith, after reflecting briefly to Jeanette that this must have been hard, continued asking questions about her family relationships. He asked her if she had experienced a difficult childhood, and Jeanette, sitting slumped in her chair, sort of chuckled and stated, "Yeah, it was miserable." Dr. Smith continued with this line of questioning, and the patient revealed that not only was she sexually abused by her father, but that her oldest child was the product of this incestuous relationship. Dr. Smith was able to ask Jeanette a couple more questions, but took his mid-session break shortly after this disclosure.

In the observation room were three behavioral science faculty and three of Dr. Smith's resident peers. During the break, Dr. Smith shared how overwhelmed he felt and stated, "I knew something was going on, but I had no idea it would be this bad. I have no idea what to do with this information." One of Dr. Smith's peers made some suggestions regarding assessing for suicidal ideation, reflecting that she may experience an increase in depression symptoms after discussing these issues. The behavioral science faculty gave clinical information regarding how disclosing traumatic experiences can make a client feel extremely vulnerable, directed Dr. Smith to ask about her support network, recommended he help her to make back-up plans for the upcoming weekend if she were to feel suicidal, and suggested referring her for psychotherapy.

Dr. Smith reentered the session, implemented all of the above suggestions, and continued to ask about her history of abuse despite his personal discomfort. He remained attuned to her cues, modifying his voice and pacing of his questions in response to hers. Toward the end of the visit, Jeanette said that she thought Dr. Smith was sent to her "by the man upstairs." Dr. Smith at first mistakenly thought she meant that a neighbor referred her to him, but on further questioning, learned that she meant that he may have been sent to her by 'God.' Dr. Smith learned that he was the first male and first physician with whom she had ever shared her full story. At the end of the session, Dr. Smith stepped out to complete some paperwork and he rejoined the patient with both the completed paperwork and a supply of a nutritional supplement from our sample closet.

In the observation room, the behavioral science faculty discussed several issues with the observing residents, all men, throughout the session. For example, issues such as exploitation, sexual abuse, and power were discussed from a feminist family systems perspective. The residents were encouraged to share their own reactions to the patient's story, how they might have conducted the session, and how their clinical care of the patient might change based on what was learned about the patient's life story.

Themes from this discussion were continued and underscored in the post-session. That is, the behavioral science faculty facilitated a discussion with Dr. Smith and his colleagues about clinical information on sexual abuse from a feminist perspective, but also emphasized Dr. Smith's use of empathy and ability to let Jeanette tell her narrative, as well as the gender and ethnic differences between them. Further discussion also centered on Dr. Smith's self-of-the-physician issues regarding his religious beliefs. Being a physician who is active in a Christian faith, he took Jeanette very seriously when she stated her belief that 'God' had sent him to her. He shared how much pressure he felt by this statement, along with feeling overwhelmed and helpless by her story. After reflecting on the session, he was able to see his offer of samples as an attempt to "do something" stemming from his sense of helplessness and his struggle with the paradigm shift away from the traditional medical stance. Dr. Smith also shared a reaction that her story was as dramatic as a movie and that he had a vision of 'popcorn flying' in the observation room as she told her story. In future practicum sessions of his own and of his colleagues, he coined the term 'popcorn moments' for such dramatic issues surfacing, hence the title of this article.

Dr. Smith has subsequently shared with us that his care of Jeanette markedly changed after this practicum session. He has been better able to integrate the biomedical and psychosocial aspects of her health, have a broad perspective and understanding of her context, and has felt more compassionate towards her. Their relationship was strengthened by this experience, and Dr. Smith takes a far more collaborative and empowering stance toward her as his patient, asking about and complimenting her on her strengths during his follow-up visits. Dr. Smith believes that he has been personally transformed by this experience and has found working with her to be rewarding.

CONCLUSION

Our perspective and supervisory methods come not only from our experiences as feminist family therapists (MED and SP) and as feminist health communication scholars (KAZ and JSK), but also may be informed by our experiences of marginalization as nonphysician women working in a largely male, patriarchal medical school. Feminist standpoint epistemology maintains that persons with less power must know not only their own culture, but also how to survive in the dominant culture, whereas the dominant group doesn't have to learn the culture of the less powerful (Harding, 1993). We are in this standpoint position as women and nonphysician faculty–trained in our own disciplines, but needing to survive within the medical education system, a system we did not personally experience as learners. This position likely highlights issues of marginalization and oppression that may be experienced by patients, residents, and women and minority faculty when interacting with a complex, patriarchal medical education and healthcare system.

Medical education has been compared to a neglectful and abusive family system because of the unrealistic expectations, denial, indirect communication patterns, rigidity, and isolation that often exist (McKegney, 1989). We attempt to provide alternative experiences based on multiple ways of knowing, being-in-relation, reflection, and use of self. Learning a being-in-relation approach and shifting power is especially important when physicians are working with medically underserved and/or marginalized patients, or those who have historically been treated paternalistically by physicians (e.g., women, ethnic minorities, gay, lesbian, or bisexual patients). As physicians learn to shift these relationships, they become agents for social change through promoting more empowering relationships.

Feminist family therapists, then, bring important lenses to medical education: a systemic conceptual framework, and an understanding of power dynamics across patients' social contexts, the doctor-patient relationship, and in the resident-faculty relationship. These combined perspectives provide a much-needed but seldom taught view of the doctor-patient relationship and complex medical systems as circular and systemic, and highlight the importance of context, understanding the patients' narrative, and the self-of-the-physician in the helping relationship.

Feminist MFTs also bring an awareness of the need for physician reflection and mindfulness of their social location, the ethical use of power, an awareness of the sociopolitical context of medicine, and the potential for physicians to be agents for social change. Both practicum as a curriculum component, and feminist supervision and teaching methods are rare in medical education. Applying the practicum training model is a good example of how feminist MFTs can not only partner with physicians, but teach essential skills while also advocating for social change through more relationship-centered, empowering physician-patient relationships.

REFERENCES

Accreditation Council for Graduate Medical Education. (2001). *Program Requirements for Residency Education in Family Practice.* Retrieved 5/13/03, http://www.acgme.org

Accreditation Council for Graduate Medical Education. (2003). *Program Requirements for Residency Education in Internal Medicine.* Retrieved 6/30/03, http://www.acgme.org

Albino, J. E., Tedesco, L. A., & Shenkle, C. L. (1990). Images of women: Reflections from the medical care system. In M. A. Paludi & G. A. Steuernagel (Eds.), *Foundations for a feminist restructuring of the academic disciplines. Haworth series on women Vol. 3* (pp. 225-253). New York: Haworth.

Ault-Riche, M. (1986). A feminist critique of 5 schools of family therapy. *The Family Therapy Collections, 16,* 1-15.

Ault-Riche, M. (1987). Teaching an integrated model of family therapy: Women as students, women as supervisors. *Journal of Psychotherapy and the Family, 3*(4), 175-192.

Avis, J. M. (1992). Where are all the family therapists? Abuse and violence within families and family therapy's response. *Journal of Marital and Family Therapy, 18,* 225-232.

Avis, J. M., & Turner, J. (1996). Feminist lenses in family therapy research: Gender, politics, and science. In D. H. Sprenkle & S. M. Moon (Eds.), *Research methods in family therapy* (pp. 145-169). New York: Guilford.

Belenky, M. F., Clinchy, B. M., Goldberger, N. R., & Tarule, J. M. (1986). *Women's ways of knowing: The development of self, voice, and mind.* New York: Basic Books.

Bograd, M. (1992). Values in conflict: Challenges to family therapists' thinking. *Journal of Marital and Family Therapy, 18,* 245-256.

Braverman, L. (1988). *Women, feminism, and family therapy.* New York: Haworth.

Bryan, L. A. (2001). Neither mask nor mirror: One therapist's journey to ethically integrate feminist family therapy and multiculturalism. *Journal of Feminist Family Therapy, 12*(2-3), 105-121.

Burge, S. K. (1991). Incorporating feminist perspectives into family medicine research. *Family Practice Research Journal, 11* (4), 349-355.

Candib, L. M. (1989). Point and counterpoint: Family life cycle theory: A feminist critique. *Family Systems Medicine, 7* (4), 473-487.

Candib, L. M. (1995). *Medicine and the family: A feminist perspective.* New York: Basic Books.

Ciamamicoli, A. P., & Ketcham, K. (2000). *The power of empathy: A practical guide to creating intimacy, self-understanding, and lasting love in your life.* New York: Dutton.

Crespi, T. D. (1995). Gender sensitive supervision: Exploring feminist perspectives for male and female supervisors. *Clinical Supervisor, 13*(2), 19-29.

Dankoski, M. E. (2000). What makes research feminist? *Journal of Feminist Family Therapy, 12*(1), 3-19.

Doherty, W. J., & Baird, M. (1983). *Family therapy and family medicine: Towards the primary care of families.* New York: Guilford.

Doherty, W. J., & Baird, M. (Eds.). (1987). *Family centered medical care: A clinical casebook.* New York: Guilford.

Doherty, W. J., Baird, M., & Becker, L. (1987). Family medicine and the biopsychosocial model: The road toward integration. *Marriage & Family Review, 10,* 51-70.

Doherty, W. J., & Campbell, T. L. (1988). *Families and health.* Thousand Oaks, CA: Sage.

Engel, G. L. (1977). The need for a new medical model: A challenge for biomedicine. *Science, 196,* 129-136.

Engel, G. L. (1980). The clinical application of the biopsychosocial model. *American Journal of Psychiatry, 137,* 535-544.

Fisher, L., & Ransom, D.C. (1997). Developing a strategy for managing behavioral healthcare within the context of primary care. *Archives of Family Medicine, 6,* 324-334.

Goldner, V. (1985). Feminism and family therapy. *Family Process, 24,* 31-47.

Goodrich, T. J., Rampage, C., Ellman, B., & Halstead, K. (1988). *Feminist family therapy: A casebook.* New York: W. W. Norton.

Hamilton, J. A. (1994). Feminist theory and health psychology: Tools for an egalitarian, woman-centered approach to women's health care. In A. J. Dan (Ed.), *Reframing women's health: Multidisciplinary research and practice* (pp. 56-66). Thousand Oaks, CA: Sage.

Harding, S. (1993). Rethinking standpoint epistemology: What is "strong objectivity"? In L. Alcoff & E. Potter (Eds.), *Feminist epistemologies* (pp. 49-82). New York: Routledge.

Hare-Mustin, R. T. (1978). A feminist approach to family therapy. *Family Process, 17,* 181-194.

Hines, P. M., Garcia Preto, N., McGoldrick, M., Almeida, R., & Weltman, S. (1999). Culture and the family life cycle. In B. Carter & M. McGoldrick (Eds.), *The expanded family life cycle: Individual, family and social perspectives* (3rd ed.). Boston: Allyn & Bacon.

Johnson, A. H. (1999). Primary care counseling. In F. C. McCutchan, D. E. Sanders, & M. E. Vogel (Eds.), *Resource guide for behavioral science educators in family medicine* (pp. 75-80). Society of Teachers of Family Medicine.

Johnson, T. W., & Colucci, P. (1999). Lesbians, gay men, and the family life cycle. In B. Carter & M. McGoldrick (Eds.), *The expanded family life cycle: Individual, family and social perspectives* (3rd ed.). Boston: Allyn & Bacon.

Jordan, J. V. (1991). Empathy and self-boundaries. In J. V. Jordan, A. G. Kaplan, J. B. Miller, I. P. Stiver, & J. L. Surrey (Eds.), *Women's growth in connection: Writings from the Stone Center* (pp. 81-96). New York: Guilford.

Kaschak, E. (Ed.). (2001). *The next generation: Third wave feminist psychotherapy.* New York: Haworth.

Kliman, J., & Madsen, W. (1999). Social class and the family life cycle. In B. Carter & M. McGoldrick (Eds.), *The expanded family life cycle: Individual, family and social perspectives* (3rd ed.). Boston: Allyn & Bacon.

Liddle, H., Davidson, G., & Barrett, M. (1988). Outcomes of live supervision: Trainee perspectives. In H. Liddle, D. Breunlin, & R. Schwartz (Eds.), *Handbook of family therapy training and supervision* (pp. 183-193). New York: Guilford.

Luepnitz, D. (1988). *The family interpreted: Feminist theory in clinical practice.* New York: Basic Books.

McDaniel, S., Campbell, T., & Seaburn, D. (1990). *Family oriented primary care: A manual for medical providers.* New York: Springer-Verlag.

McDaniel, S., Campbell, T., Wynne, L., & Weber, T. (1988). Family systems consultation: Opportunities for teaching in family medicine. *Family Systems Medicine, 6,* 391-403.

McDaniel, S. H., Hepworth, J., & Doherty, W. J. (1992). *Medical family therapy: A biopsychosocial approach to families with health problems.* New York: Basic Books.

McGoldrick, M. (Ed.). (1998). *Revisioning family therapy: Race, gender and culture in clinical practice.* New York: Guilford.

McKegney, C. P. (1989). Medical education: A neglectful and abusive family system. *Family Medicine, 21,* 452-457.

Mirkin, M. P. (Ed.). (1990). *The social and political contexts of family therapy.* Boston: Allyn & Bacon.

Mirkin, M. P. (Ed.). (1994). *Women in context: Toward a feminist reconstruction of psychotherapy.* New York: Guilford.

Montalvo, B., & Storm, C. L. (1997). Live supervision revolutionizes the supervision process. In T. C. Todd, & C. L. Storm (Eds.), *The complete systemic supervisor* (pp. 283-297). Boston: Allyn & Bacon.

Patterson, J., Bischoff, R. J., & McIntosh-Koontz, L. (1998). Training issues in integrated care. In A. Blount (Ed.), *Integrated primary care: The future of medical and mental health collaboration* (pp. 261-283). New York: Norton.

Patterson, J., Peek, C. J., Heinrich, R. L., Bischoff, R. J., & Scherger, J. (2002). *Mental health professionals in medical settings: A primer.* New York: Norton.

Patterson, J., Scherger, J., Bischoff, R. J., & McIntosh-Koontz, L. (1998). Training for collaboration: Suggestions for the joint training of mental health clinicians and family practice residents. *Families, Systems & Health, 16*(1-2), 147-157.

Porter, N., Vasquez, M., Fygetakis, L., Mangione, L., Nickerson, E. T., Pieniadz, J. et al. (1997). Covision: Feminist supervision, process, and collaboration. In J. Worell & N. G. Johnson (Eds.), *Shaping the future of feminist psychology: Education, research, & practice. Psychology of women book series* (pp. 155-171). Washington, DC: American Psychological Association.

Prouty, A. (2001). Experiencing feminist family therapy supervision. *Journal of Feminist Family Therapy, 12*(4), 171-203.

Prouty, A. M., & Bermudez, M. J. (1999). Experiencing multiconsciousness: A feminist model for therapy. *Journal of Feminist Family Therapy, 11*(3), 19-39.

Prouty, A. M., Thomas, V., Johnson, S., & Long, J. K. (2001). Methods of feminist family therapy supervision. *Journal of Marital and Family Therapy, 27*, 85-97.

Ruzek, S. B. (1978). *The women's health movement: Feminist alternatives to medical control.* New York: Praeger.

Scheingold, L. (1988). Balint work in England: Lessons for American family medicine. *Journal of Family Practice, 26*(3), 315-320.

Seaburn, D. B., Lorenz, A. D., Gunn, W. B., Gawinski, B. A., & Mauksch, L. B. (1996). *Models of collaboration: A guide for mental health professionals working with health care practitioners.* New York: Basic Books.

Taggart, M. (1985). The feminist critique in epistemological perspective: Questions of context in family therapy. *Journal of Marital and Family Therapy, 11*, 113-126.

Walter, C. A. (1988). The dilemma of the female physician in the feminist health center. *Journal of the American Medical Women's Association, 43*, 45-50.

Walters, M., Carter, B., Papp, P., & Silverstein, O. (1988). *The invisible web: Gender patterns in family relationships.* New York: Guilford.

Weingarten, K., & Bograd, M. L. (Eds.). (1996). *Reflections on feminist family therapy training.* New York: Haworth.

Wheeler, D., Avis, J.M., Miller, L. A., & Chaney, S. (1985). Rethinking family therapy education and supervision: A feminist model. *Journal of Psychotherapy and the Family, 1*(4), 53-71.

Wright, C. I., & Fish, L. S. (1997). Feminist family therapy: The battle against subtle sexism. In N. V. Benokraitis (Ed.), *Subtle sexism: Current practice and prospects for change* (pp. 201-215). Thousand Oaks, CA: Sage.

A "Golden Girl" Tarnished: Amplifying One Patient's (and Family's) Voice Through Collaborative Care in a Family Medicine Setting

Todd M. Edwards
Jo Ellen Patterson

SUMMARY. Medical family therapy has become a popular specialization in family therapy, resulting in more and more clinicians pursuing clinical opportunities in primary and tertiary care. We believe it is important for family therapists to understand the differences between medical settings, particularly the diversity in patient presentations. The purpose of this paper is to present some unique characteristics of mental health services in family medicine. Because family physicians are often the first contact for someone coping with a mental health and/or family concern, they provide emotional support and direction to mental health services. A case example helps illustrate a common patient presentation in family medicine and the role family therapists can play in providing mental

Todd M. Edwards, PhD, is Associate Professor and Director, Marital and Family Therapy Program, School of Education, University of San Diego, 5998 Alcala Park, San Diego, CA 92110 (E-mail: tedwards@sandiego.edu).

Jo Ellen Patterson, PhD, is Professor, Marital and Family Therapy Program, School of Education, University of San Diego, 5998 Alcala Park, San Diego, CA 92110 (E-mail: joellen@sandiego.edu).

[Haworth co-indexing entry note]: "A 'Golden Girl' Tarnished: Amplifying One Patient's (and Family's) Voice Through Collaborative Care in a Family Medicine Setting." Edwards, Todd M., and Jo Ellen Patterson. Co-published simultaneously in *Journal of Feminist Family Therapy* (The Haworth Press, Inc.) Vol. 15, No. 2/3, 2003, pp. 75-88; and: *Feminist Perspectives in Medical Family Therapy* (ed: Anne M. Prouty Lyness) The Haworth Press, Inc., 2003. pp. 75-88. Single or multiple copies of this article are available for a fee from The Haworth Document Delivery Service [1-800-HAWORTH, 9:00 a.m. - 5:00 p.m. (EST). E-mail address: docdelivery@haworthpress.com].

Digital Object Identifier: 10.1300/J086v15n02_04

health services to patients and family members in a family medicine set- ting. *[Article copies available for a fee from The Haworth Document Delivery Service: 1-800-HAWORTH. E-mail address: <docdelivery@haworthpress.com> Website: <http://www.HaworthPress.com> © 2003 by The Haworth Press, Inc. All rights reserved.]*

KEYWORDS. Medical family therapy, collaboration, family medicine, family therapy

Medical family therapy (McDaniel, Hepworth, & Doherty, 1992) has garnered tremendous attention in the field of family therapy over the past decade. What started as an interest for a handful of prominent fam- ily therapists has blossomed into a full-blown specialty, evidenced by the creation of several medical family therapy internships and a recent pro- posal to establish the first doctoral program in medical family therapy at East Carolina University. Family therapy's heightened interest in medi- cine is timely as health care shifts toward a greater emphasis on collabo- rative care. With its relational approach to mental health services, family therapy is well positioned to play a key role in the rapidly changing health care environment.

Although the label medical family therapy has been helpful in captur- ing the work of family therapists in medical settings and has unified many therapists working in medical settings, it has, at times, hidden the diver- sity in medical settings. In other words, different medical settings pres- ent unique challenges and obstacles and demand a variety of therapeutic skills. When my (TE) interest in medical settings surfaced and I began pur- suing training opportunities, I thought that I would be helping families cope with a wide range of chronic illnesses. If my training experiences had taken place with cancer patients in oncology or with Type 1 diabet- ics in Endocrinology, my assumptions would have been correct. Instead, my training took place in family medicine, which meant working with pa- tients, families, and physicians in conversation about depression, anxi- ety, chronic pain, relationship issues, and/or problems that often lacked specificity.

Articulating the full range of the differences in family therapy in medi- cine goes beyond the scope of this paper. We want to share the challenges and rewards of working in a family medicine setting. We chose to focus on family medicine because of our years of experience in primary care and our belief that most medical family therapists will find a home in family medicine. As any family physician will attest to, there is a tremendous need for mental health services in family medicine clinics. Family therapists also share similar values as family physicians, most notably an interest in systems thinking, family competence, and preventative interventions.

Some of the unique characteristics of providing family therapy in family medicine include an awareness of outpatient medical culture, sharing care with professionals from multiple disciplines, and understanding a wide range of physical concerns that are sometimes vague and difficult to understand (Edwards, 2002; Gawinski, Edwards, & Speice, 1999; McDaniel et al., 1992). Many patients seen in outpatient family medicine clinics have not had previous access to mental health services, do not know they have access to mental health services, or are hesitant to pursue mental health services due to the stigma of seeing a mental health professional or to previous negative experiences with the mental health community. In our family medicine setting, we see many patients who choose to seek mental health services because their family physician recommends it and it is offered in the same location as the medical services. The case example presented in this paper tells the story of a woman who had a variety of physical problems that could not be defined. She was continually shuttled to psychiatry, perpetuating a mind-body split that made her feel stigmatized and marginalized. Our on-site collaborative model attempted to rectify this injustice.

In the following section, we describe the culture of family medicine followed by an overview of collaboration among professionals in family medicine. Following the overview of collaboration, we present one treatment model used in the care of one patient and her family. We conclude with reflections on the patient and her family and the overall benefits of providing mental health services in family medicine.

THE CULTURE OF FAMILY MEDICINE

Family medicine began as a distinct specialty almost fifty years ago. Before the existence of family medicine, patients were treated by their general practitioner. In the United States, the primary distinction between general practice and family practice is that family practice physicians complete a three-year residency that includes some hospital-based training. In addition, family practice physicians must pass board certification exams in addition to state licensing exams.

Family physicians have always seen mental health care as part of their treatment scope along with the more traditional physical illnesses. A position paper from the American Academy of Family Physicians states the following:

> Family physicians are trained specifically to provide mental health services, which are an essential component of comprehensive primary medical care. Patients frequently seek care from their primary care physicians for symptomatic complaints with underlying psycho-social problems. (American Academy of Family Physicians, 1994, p. 1)

Although intense demands on their time often make it difficult for family physicians to treat the whole patient, including addressing mental health concerns, patients look to their doctors for mental health care. In fact, research suggests that primary care is the de facto mental health system (McDaniel, Campbell, & Seaburn, 1995; Patterson, Peek, Heinrich, Bischoff, & Scherger, 2002; Regier, Goldberg, & Taube, 1978). In other words, if people seek care for mental health concerns, they are most likely to seek treatment from their physician, not a mental health specialist (Patterson et al., 2002).

When a patient who is depressed, anxious, and/or has a family problem goes to see her family physician, she may not report depression, anxiety or family problem on her intake questionnaire. Instead, she may report difficulty sleeping, headaches, or low energy. It is left to the physician to decipher what these symptoms mean. Research suggests that approximately half of all patients seeing their family physician have some mental health concern (Chudy & Dea, 1996; Pincus, Tanielian, Marcus, Olfson, Zarin, Thompson, & Zito, 1998; Regier, Narrow, Rae, Manderscheid, Locke, & Goodwin, 1993; Strosahl, 1997). These mental health concerns may be obvious to the patient and physician, hidden from the physician with patient awareness, or elude awareness by both physician and patient. At times, a family member is a resource in raising awareness of mental health concerns.

In general, family medicine settings provide patients and their families with an avenue to mental health services when it is likely patients would never seek out mental health care on their own (Reust, Thomlinson, & Lattie, 1999). Most people have some access to medical care but might not have access to mental health care. Marginalized people such as minorities, the elderly, the unemployed, and the disabled usually have access to some type of medical care.

In contrast, few people have access to or use professional mental health services. As a result, patients who enter mental health services co-located in their physician's office have often never seen a mental health professional before, nor were they seeking mental health services when they visited their family physician's office. For the first time, many patients have access to mental health providers and vice versa.

FAMILY MEDICINE-FAMILY THERAPY COLLABORATION

The early leaders of family medicine shared many of the same ideals as family therapists. They wanted to treat entire families and viewed patients as members of families, not simply individuals. They intended to provide holistic care that included prevention and education, not simply treating illnesses. Similar to family therapists, family physicians focus on patients' strengths, context, and the doctor-patient relationship.

When the physician, patient, and/or family members are able to identify a mental health concern or a physician believes a patient would benefit from mental health services, the shared values and commitment to family-centered care make family medicine an ideal setting for collaboration between family therapists and family physicians. When patients report vague symptoms, the physician and family therapist together can assess the patient's needs and create a treatment plan, which often includes family members. Seaburn, Gawinski, Harp, McDaniel, Waxman, and Shields (1993) provide an excellent example of this collaborative model in the family medicine residency program at the University of Rochester.

Faculty in the Marital and Family Therapy (MFT) program at the University of San Diego (USD) currently provide MFT training and resident education in the family medicine residency at the University of California in San Diego (UCSD). The family medicine residency is the clinical and educational arm of the UCSD Department of Family and Community Medicine. Graduates from the USD MFT program provide low-fee mental health services to patients within the clinic and are trained alongside family medicine residents in a collaborative model.

Our on-site mental health services operate in a similar way as many other collaborative care practices. Counseling is available to patients who are members of the medical practice. Referrals to our MFT interns come from residents in training to become family physicians, faculty physicians, and nurse practitioners. Similar to Seaburn et al. (1993), a typical patient in our practice is a single mother in her 30s with multiple psychosocial and medical problems, such as depression, anxiety, and relationship problems.

Therapists who are successful in our clinic have some respect for a biomedical model and medical language. This does not mean that they exclude systems thinking, rather, they adopt a biopsychosocial, systems model (Engel, 1977). The therapists also are assertive enough to develop close, ongoing relationships with their physician colleagues. Successful management of this relationship, which is characterized by mutual respect, ongoing communication, and the development of a common mission (McDaniel, Campbell, & Seaburn, 1995), contributes to a positive clinical outcome.

An additional key to success is gaining comfort with the nontraditional role of a family therapist in family medicine. Family therapists in family medicine often intervene in diverse ways. For example, an immediate crisis may require acute psychosocial consultation followed by a referral elsewhere or the establishment of a short-term treatment plan to stabilize a patient with the assistance of a family and extrafamilial support system. Most patients referred to mental health services are seen in ongoing therapy, but family therapists in family medicine need to define their role with as much flexibility as possible.

Joint Training

One of the unique features of our setting is the joint training of family medicine residents and family therapists. The Behavioral Health (BH) Clinic, which is very similar to live supervision in family therapy, is one teaching method that formally brings these students together. The clinic is structured as follows: A family therapy intern and/or a family medicine resident invites a patient to the afternoon clinic in order to obtain feedback from a multidisciplinary group of health care professionals, which includes family medicine residents, a psychiatrist, a licensed family therapist, and a family therapy intern.[1] Referrals are made to the clinic for a variety of concerns such as depression, anxiety, substance abuse, medication management, relationship distress, and coping with chronic pain and illness.

When patients and their families are referred to the behavioral health clinic, this is not the first time they have been seen by a medical or mental health provider in our office. It is a moment in the course of their illness where a team of providers reflects on what is presented and provides direction to the patient, family, and referring therapist or physician. Students who are seeking another perspective on a challenging patient commonly make referrals. Details about the structure of the clinic have been described elsewhere (Edwards, Patterson, Grauf-Grounds, & Groban, 2001).

THE BEHAVIORAL HEALTH CLINIC IN ACTION

"The Golden Girl" and Her Father

A family medicine resident referred Tamara, a 41-year-old Caucasian woman, to the Behavioral Health Clinic for multiple medical problems, including Tourette's Syndrome, a pituitary gland tumor, hair loss, muscle mass loss, multiple head injuries, and many other concerns. Tamara, appearing thin and fragile, arrived at the interview accompanied by her father, Jim, a tall, husky 60-year-old Caucasian man with a booming voice. For this particular patient, one of the family therapy interns joined the resident in the interview.

Upon walking in the exam room, Jim stated why he accompanied Tamara to the interview and requested an opportunity to read his prepared statement about Tamara's health problems. He described the physical and psychological changes he had seen in Tamara over the past several years and concluded that she has "a complex aggregate of symptoms that eludes diagnosis by specialists." Jim expressed frustration and disenchantment with a trap that had felt inescapable: "A diagnosis for Tamara is elusive, her symptoms are assumed to be 'psychosomatic,' and she is continually referred to psychiatrists who do not know how to help her."

Tamara is the younger of two daughters. According to Jim, she was the "golden girl." For example, he provided a list of her many accomplishments: high school honor roll, senior class president, participant in multiple high school sports, college dean's list, college athletics, beautiful, and extremely bright, with an IQ of 160. Jim stated, "This is not the lifestyle we had envisioned [for her]."

Tamara declared that she was a picture of good health until 1993. In 1993, she experienced Rheumatoid Fever, which began an onslaught of medical problems that progressively worsened. After little success with multiple specialists, including several neurologists and endocrinologists, she echoed her father's frustration with the medical system's inability to provide her with an accurate diagnosis. Tamara sincerely believed that she had a serious illness that was slowly killing her and that the medical system was failing her by its inability to hear her concerns.

The following exchange between the MFT intern and Tamara captures Tamara's desperation:

> MFT: Is there something you would like us to know or share with us today?

> Tamara: I have a chip on my shoulder when it comes to doctors, with good reason. Due to my level of frustration and physical pain, I tend to speak with venomous tones sometimes. I don't mean to direct this at you, but. . . . My foremost need is someone who can see me regularly. If someone can't see me regularly, then please let me know now . . . I really believe that I have a disease process that is literally killing me before your eyes, but every specialist I've seen conducts a few traditional surface tests that are inconsistent [and inconclusive], which makes them conclude that there is nothing wrong with me. Each of these isolated specialists cannot put their finger on any consistent specific pathology in their specialization, especially in one appointment, so they conclude it's psychological. I want a primary care physician that looks at me globally, currently, and historically to see the physical degradation over time and make some medical sense of it. Just because some medical personnel are stumped doesn't mean nothing is wrong with me. I want a doctor who is interested and willing to be thorough, non-confrontational, and open-minded.

> MFT: Basically you want someone who will listen to you, not make premature judgments, and show you that they care.

> Tamara: Exactly. I want someone to really listen.

After a 20-minute interview, the MFT intern and family medicine resident excused themselves and consulted with the team.

The Collaborative Care Team's Response

The team included the intern and resident who conducted the interview, a psychiatrist, a family therapist, and a 4th year medical student. The team agreed that Tamara and her family were burdened by many physical concerns. However, what was also troubling was her sense of marginalization in the medical culture. Even with presumably well-intentioned medical providers, Tamara believed her voice had not been heard, and she was repeatedly jettisoned from specialist to specialist because no one could find a firm diagnosis. As time progressed, Tamara's rage increased, which was communicated to medical providers who found her to be a difficult patient, which further complicated her care. Both the resident and family therapy intern experienced her as extremely challenging.

Our primary goal in this consultation was to *not* repeat her previous experiences in the medical system. Although it had been partially repeated through the referral to our Behavioral Health Clinic, we did not want her and her father to walk away with a similar conclusion. Tamara saw herself as a woman whose body was slowly deteriorating and her presence progressively erased, making it harder and harder for her voice to be heard. The fact that she did not have one central, trustworthy, consistent person who could manage her care and the treatment team made her feel invisible in the medical community. From Tamara's perspective, she was a problem that kept getting moved from physician to physician, with no one taking responsibility for her health care.

Tamara requested consistent, frequent patient care in order to develop a clear understanding of her physical concerns. We agreed with her assessment. However, we added another component. Our recommendation was that Tamara could be seen by the resident physician for 6 successive weeks in order to more fully understand her physical concerns and do the necessary work-up to determine the correct diagnoses and treatment plan. In addition, Tamara, and her family if possible, could meet with the MFT intern during the hour prior to her medical visit to review the previous week, organize her concerns for the medical visit, and discuss any other relevant issues. This hour was not framed as therapy. Rather, the family therapy intern would serve as her "health care counselor"[2] and would work in close collaboration with the resident and other consulting physicians to ensure that her voice was being heard. Our hope was that once a relationship developed between Tamara, her family, and the MFT intern, she would eventually be willing to talk about how the medical problems affect her and her family and how stress might exacerbate some of her medical problems.

The Family's Response

Tamara's father responded to the team's feedback with great enthusiasm. Tamara, in contrast, was highly suspicious and lobbied for an intervention that would involve the assignment of someone as her ombudsman or full-time health care advocate. The physician and family therapist listened attentively, empathized with her frustration and anger and assured her that her concerns would be addressed using the suggested approach. They also assured her that the old approach of "evaluate and refer out" would not occur. Rather, the on-site health care team would work with her to provide integrated treatment, allowing the range of her concerns to be heard and addressed in one place. Tamara underscored the urgency of her situation but agreed to try this approach.

The Preliminary Outcome

The MFT intern met with Tamara both individually and with her parents for several sessions. Based on the treatment suggestions of McDaniel et al. (1992), the initial emphasis of the work was placed on joining, which was facilitated by accepting Tamara's definition of the problem rather than quickly shifting the focus to psychosocial issues and emotional reframes. In addition to joining, the MFT intern embraced the uncertainty surrounding the situation and recruited Tamara's family, particularly her father, to serve as consultants to facilitate a better understanding of what makes the problems better and worse. There also was an emphasis on Tamara's survival skills that enabled her to get through the trauma of the past 10 years (White, 1995).

During these sessions, it became apparent that Tamara was having continued difficulty with her resident physician. She was confident in the resident's competence but knew that the resident would eventually finish her training and transfer her to another physician. As a part of their ongoing collaboration, the MFT intern and resident had several discussions about the progress of treatment and the resident expressed similar concerns about Tamara's inability to trust her. Tamara had ongoing interactions with the resident's supervising physician and told the MFT intern that she felt very comfortable with his gentleness, competence, and stability at the clinic. The intern and resident decided to talk with the supervising physician about his ability to see her and then jointly met with Tamara to offer a transfer to the supervising physician. The supervising physician began seeing Tamara on a regular basis and significant progress was made. Her physical problems did not disappear, but for the first time she felt acknowledged and validated, partly due to the relationship with her new doctor and partly due to the close collaborative relationship between her doctor and the MFT intern. She had never experienced a time when her health care providers were truly in meaningful conversation with one another. More importantly, they were talking *with* her rather than *to* her.

REFLECTIONS

When patients present with a variety of symptoms that defy medical explanation, sometimes referred to as a Somatoform Disorder (DSM-IV-TR, 2000), the patient, family members, and physicians can struggle with feelings of helplessness, anger and despair. According to Griffith and Griffith (1994), these emotions can lead to conflict and resentment in the doctor-patient relationship:

> When clinicians cannot find solutions for mind-body problems, then the patients and their families genuinely suffer from the symptoms that continue unabated. This failure exacts yet another toll when frustrated clinicians and patients reach for a target to blame. The temptation for clinician and patient to accuse each other of bad faith is nearly irresistible. (p. 11)

Tamara and her physicians became engaged in a negative physician-patient interaction (McDaniel, Campbell, & Seaburn, 1990). Her original primary care physician focused on her biomedical symptoms, referred her to specialists, tests were negative (leaving Tamara confused), her physicians then focused on psychosocial stress and referred her to psychiatrists, Tamara felt angry and misunderstood and requested more tests, physicians withdrew or referred to more specialists, Tamara initiated a search for new physicians, and the cycle was continuing.

Like many patients in similar situations, Tamara felt disqualified and without a voice in her health care. Unfortunately, such silence has been a common experience for women interacting with many larger systems, particularly health care systems (Imber-Black, 1991). This was extremely painful for her and her family. The last thing we wanted to see happen with Tamara and her father was for them to walk away with another painful, hollow experience with health care professionals. We wanted to amplify her voice with the hope of finding the intersection between her mental health and physical concerns. Her physical concerns were not simply an expression of mental illness. Rather, her physical concerns had a stressful effect on her mood, behavior, and relationships and ongoing stress complicated her physical concerns. Never did we believe that her symptoms were "all in her head," but that is the message that some patients like Tamara receive during health care interactions with well-intentioned physicians.

Her situation was in desperate need of a team approach that included a medical family therapist. Close, on-site collaboration between health care providers had the potential to help heal the mind-body split that was so damaging to Tamara in her treatment history. Both the therapist and the physician could contribute to a holistic, context-sensitive view of the Tamara's problems and create a more comprehensive treatment plan. Even though previous referrals to psychiatrists were unhelpful, including a psychiatrist on the collaborative team could be very helpful. We believe that this kind of integrated treatment helps honor the patient's voice because collaboration emphasizes a partnership with the patient and family as opposed to a traditional hierarchical relationship that can be so silencing (McDaniel et al., 1992).

The MFT intern's role in the case of Tamara is typical in a family medicine setting. In collaborative care, the therapist's responsibility is not simply to provide direct service to the patient. Instead, the therapist is a significant support person to the patient's physician. Compared to a traditional therapist, the medical family therapist expands her treatment focus. The patient, the patient's family, the physician, and the medical setting are all areas of concern for the medical family therapist.

In addition, the care plan may be shorter, longer, or completely different than the usual therapy treatment (e.g., weekly 50-minute sessions over three months). Flexibility and tailoring the treatment plan to the individual patient's and family's needs are key hallmarks of medical family therapy. In Tamara's case, the typical treatments of psychotropic medications or referral to a specialist were eschewed for a tailor-made plan that incorporated her specific beliefs and requests about her care.

CONCLUSION

We hope that the ideas presented in this paper provide clinicians new to medical family therapy with new knowledge about the unique qualities and opportunities in a family medicine setting. Family medicine is a culture full of ambiguity and complexity, mostly due to the intricate interaction between mental health and physical health, which can test the patience of physicians, patients, and family members. Co-locating mental health services in family medicine can help to decrease this frustration and build a bridge between health care providers, patients, and families to insure optimal care for *everyone*.

NOTES

1. In California, an MFT intern refers to someone who has completed a master's degree in MFT and is working towards MFT licensure.
2. We borrowed this label from Drs. Susan McDaniel and Tom Campbell, who used "health care counselors" in their study of collaborative care for high utilizers of medical care.

REFERENCES

Americian Academy of Family Physicians. (1994). *White paper on the provision of mental health care services by family physicians.* Kansas City, MO: Author.

American Psychiatric Association. (2000). *Diagnostic and statistical manual of mental disorders: Text revision* (4th ed.). Washington, DC: Author.

Chudy, J. H., & Dea, R. A. (1996, March). *Integrating behavioral healthcare and primary care.* Paper presented at the meeting of the Primary Care Behavioral Healthcare Summit, San Diego, CA.

DeGruy, F. (1997). Mental healthcare in the primary care setting: A paradigm problem. *Families, Systems & Health, 15,* 3-26.

Edwards, T. M. (2002). *Essential skills in medical family therapy supervision.* Poster session presented at the American Association for Marriage and Family Therapy Annual Conference, Cincinnati, OH.

Edwards, T. M., Patterson, J., Grauf-Grounds, C., & Groban, S. (2001). Psychiatry, MFT, & family medicine collaboration: The Sharp behavioral health clinic. *Families, Systems & Health, 19,* 25-36.

Engel, G. (1977). The need for a new medical model: A challenge for biomedicine. *Science, 196,* 129-136.

Gawinski, B. A., Edwards, T. M., & Speice, J. (1999). A family therapy internship in a multidisciplinary health care setting: Trainees' and supervisor's reflections. *Journal of Marital and Family Therapy, 25,* 469-484.

Griffith, J. L., & Griffith, M. E. (1994). *The body speaks: Therapeutic dialogues for mind-body problems.* New York: Basic Books.

Imber-Black, E. (1991). Women's relationships with larger systems. In M. McGoldrick, C. M. Anderson, & F. Walsh (Eds.), *Women in families: A framework for family therapy.* New York: Norton.

McDaniel, S., Campbell, T., & Seaburn, D. (1990). *Family-oriented primary care: A manual for medical providers.* New York: Springer-Verlag.

McDaniel, S. H., Campbell, T. L., & Seaburn, D. B. (1995). Principles of collaboration between health and mental health providers in primary care. *Families, Systems & Health, 13,* 283-299.

McDaniel, S. H., Hepworth, J., & Doherty, W. J. (1992). *Medical family therapy: A biopsychosocial approach to families with health problems.* New York: Basic Books.

Patterson, J., Peek, C. J., Heinrich, R. L., Bischoff, R., & Scherger, J. E. (2002). *Mental health professionals in medical settings: A primer.* New York: Norton.

Pincus, H. A., Tanielian, T. L., Marcus, S. C., Olfson, M., Zarin, D. A., Thompson, J., & Zito, J. M. (1998). Prescribing trends in psychotropic medications. *Journal of the American Medical Association, 279,* 526-531.

Regier, D. A., Goldberg, I. D., & Taube, C. A. (1978). The de facto US mental health services system. *Archives of General Psychiatry, 35,* 685-693.

Regier, D. A., Narrow, W. E., Rae, D. S., Manderscheid, R. W., Locke, B. Z., & Goodwin, F. K. (1993). The de facto U.S. mental and addictive disorders service system: Epidemiologic catchment area prospective 1-year prevalence rates of disorder and services. *Archives of General Psychiatry, 50,* 85-94.

Reust, C. E., Thomlinson, R. P., & Lattie, D. (1999). Keeping or missing the initial behavioral health appointment; A qualitative study of referrals in a primary care setting. *Families, Systems & Health, 17,* 399-411.

Seaburn, D., Gawinski, B., Harp, J., McDaniel, S., Waxman, D., & Shields, C. (1993). Family systems therapy in a primary care medical setting: The Rochester experience. *Journal of Marital and Family Therapy, 19,* 177-190.

Seaburn, D. B., Lorenz, A. D., Gunn, W. B., Gawinski, B. A., & Mauksch, L. B. (1996). *Models of collaboration: A guide for mental health professionals working with health care practitioners.* New York: Basic Books.

Strosahl, K. (1997). Building primary care behavioral health systems that work: A compass and a horizon. In N. A. Cummings, J. L. Cummings, & J. N. Johnson (Eds.), *Behavioral health in primary care: A guide for clinical integration* (pp. 37-60). Madison, CT: Psychosocial Press.

White, M. (1995). *Re-authoring lives: Interviews & essays.* Adelaide, South Australia: Dulwich Centre.

Vulvar Vestibulitis Syndrome: Therapeutic Implications for Couples

Jennifer Connor

SUMMARY. The author examines vulvar vestibulitis syndrome, a women's health condition that is rarely discussed in family therapy literature. An argument is made regarding the relevancy to couple therapists. A review of diagnosis, prevalence rates, and treatment is provided. The empirical research findings for psychological, interpersonal, and sexual correlates are presented, and implications for couple therapists are discussed. *[Article copies available for a fee from The Haworth Document Delivery Service: 1-800-HAWORTH. E-mail address: <docdelivery@haworthpress.com> Website: <http://www.HaworthPress.com> © 2003 by The Haworth Press, Inc. All rights reserved.]*

KEYWORDS. Vulvar vestibulitis, couple therapy, feminist psychotherapy, sex therapy, medical family therapy, women's health

Jennifer Connor, MS, is a doctoral candidate in the Department of Family Social Science at the University of Minnesota Twin Cities.

Address correspondence to: Jennifer Connor, 290 McNeal Hall, 1985 Buford Avenue, St. Paul, MN 55108 (E-mail: jconnor@che.umn.edu).

The author would like to thank Jim Maddock for his comments on an earlier edition of this paper. His dedication to his students is truly appreciated.

[Haworth co-indexing entry note]: "Vulvar Vestibulitis Syndrome: Therapeutic Implications for Couples." Connor, Jennifer. Co-published simultaneously in *Journal of Feminist Family Therapy* (The Haworth Press, Inc.) Vol. 15, No. 2/3, 2003, pp. 89-98; and: *Feminist Perspectives in Medical Family Therapy* (ed: Anne M. Prouty Lyness) The Haworth Press, Inc., 2003, pp. 89-98. Single or multiple copies of this article are available for a fee from The Haworth Document Delivery Service [1-800-HAWORTH, 9:00 a.m. - 5:00 p.m. (EST). E-mail address: docdelivery@haworthpress.com].

Digital Object Identifier: 10.1300/J086v15n02_05

Often when I tell other couple and family therapists that I am interested in women's health issues, especially vulvar vestibulitis, they look slightly confused and remark that they have never heard of vulvar vestibulitis. Yet, as this paper will demonstrate, vulvar vestibulitis is not rare, and it especially influences a couple's sexual experiences. Because a couple's sexual experiences are an important component of most couples' relationships, it is my conviction that couple therapists should be aware of this syndrome and its impact on women and couples' lives. When therapists remain ignorant of health issues particular to women, a disservice is done to women who are in both physical and psychological pain. The intent of this paper is to provide an introduction to what is known about the symptoms, etiology, and treatment of the vulvar vestibulitis syndrome. A review of the research describing the psychological, relational, and sexual states of women with vulvar vestibulitis syndrome will be provided. Finally, the clinical implications for couple therapists will be discussed.

WHAT DO WE KNOW ABOUT VULVAR VESTIBULITIS?

Vulvar vestibulitis is a pain disorder of the vulva and falls under the broader classification of vulvodynia (Byth, 1998). Reports of the symptoms of vulvar vestibulitis have been present in the literature for over a hundred years (Byth, 1998). However, the disorder did not receive a name until 1987, when Friedrich described the criteria for the diagnosis (Friedrich, 1987). For women with vulvar vestibulitis, pain is experienced when pressure is placed on the vulvar vestibule (Byth, 1998). Activities that may induce pain include vaginal intercourse, tampon use, and gynecological examinations (Bergeron, Binik, Khalife, & Pagidas, 1997). Women also complain of postcoital burning (Bergeron et al., 1997b). Some women report that wearing tight pants or underwear made of certain fabrics can be uncomfortable (Schover, Youngs, & Cannata, 1992). A diagnosis can be made during a gynecological examination in which the gynecologist is able to determine that the pain is localized in the vulvar vestibular glands (Bergeron et al., 1997b).

Many articles cite Goetsch (1991) when reporting prevalence rates. Goetsch reported that 15% of her sample in a gynecological clinic met the criteria of vulvar vestibulitis. However, the sample consisted of 210 women, eight of whom were not Caucasian. Epidemiological studies need to be done with a heterogeneous sample in order to determine prevalence rates. Additionally, many report that vulvar vestibulitis is primarily found in Caucasian women; however, this may also need further invest-igation. Mistakes have been made in the past when suggesting that a disease was only prevalent in Caucasian women. For example, endo-metriosis was considered a white middle class woman's disease, but now it is known that women of many backgrounds suffer with endo-metriosis (Weinstein, 1988). It is evident that further epidemiological studies need to be completed in order to define the demographic risk factors of vulvar vestibulitis.

The etiology of vulvar vestibulitis is unclear, as is the best approach to treatment. Many women describe going to multiple doctors before re-ceiving a diagnosis and subsequently trying many different treatments, often with poor results (Bergeron et al., 1997b). Possible causes that have been investigated include multiple candidiasis infections, use of antifungal or prescribed vaginal creams, allergies, human papillomavirus, hormonal factors, and a history of urinary tract infections (Bergeron et al., 1997b). Another possibility proposed by dermatologists is that vul-var vestibulitis is a dermatological condition (O'Hare & Sherertz, 2000). It has also been argued that vulvar vestibulitis is a multidimensional pain disorder, meaning that medical factors may interact with psycho-social processes (Bergeron, Binik, Khalife, Meana, Berkley, & Pagidas, 1997).

TREATMENT

Most gynecologists have attempted to use the least invasive treatments first, but some have performed surgery when other forms of treatment have failed. Bergeron et al. (1997b) reported that surgery has been in-vestigated more frequently than other treatments, and has the most con-sistent positive results. Two types of surgeries have been investigated, vestibulectomies and laser treatments. A vestibulectomy "consists of an excision of the hymen and of all the sensitive areas of the vestibule, most frequently located in the posterior fourchette, to a depth of ~2 mm. The vaginal mucosa is then mobilized and brought downward to cover the excised area" (Bergeron et al., 1997b, p. 32). Schover et al. (1992) reported successfully using a similar surgery, without the removal of the hymen. Reid et al. (1995) investigated using flashlamp-excited dye laser therapy for women with vulvar vestibulitis, and demonstrated that it is both safe and effective. Other treatments that have demonstrated some efficacy include lidocaine jelly (for mild cases), intralesional alpha interferon injections, low doses of amitriptyline, behavior and sex therapy, and biofeedback (Bergeron et al., 1997b).

PSYCHOSOCIAL RESEARCH

Psychological Factors

Several researchers have explored the psychological features of women with vulvar vestibulitis. All studies have been cross-sectional, and therefore it is impossible to determine if any psychological difficulties demonstrated by subjects were present previous to the onset of vulvar vestibulitis. Additionally, findings have been contradictory; therefore it is unclear whether or not women with vulvar vestibulitis differ from the general population. It may be that when and how the women were assessed has contributed to the discrepancies in research results.

Meana, Binik, Khalife, and Cohen (1997) reported that although women with dyspareunia reported more psychopathology than women in a comparison group, when women were separated into subgroups, those with vulvar vestibulitis did not differ from the women in the comparison group on amount of psychopathology. Schover et al. (1992) found that women in their sample did not differ from normed data on standardized questionnaires measuring depression, somatization or anxiety. However, Schover et al. report that when measuring depression through a standardized interview, women with vulvar vestibulitis reported a significantly higher level of depression. Van Lankveld, Weijenborg, and Ter Kuile (1996) also reported that women in their sample did not differ from women in a comparison group on psychopathology and psychological distress. However, there was a significant difference between groups on shyness and somatization. Jantos and White (1997) provided contrary evidence. Women in their sample scored high on measures for depression, anxiety, suicidal ideation, and perfectionistic traits. Gates and Galask (2001) also found that women with vulvar vestibulitis in their sample reported higher depression and psychological distress than women in a comparison group.

Overall it would appear that women in many samples are in some distress. However, as stated above, it cannot be determined if distress or psychological symptoms are the result of living with a disorder, contributed to the origins or maintenance of the disorder, or related to other aspects of the women's lives. Many may be quick to assume that genital pain in women is related to previous abuse; however, research has indicated that women within the categorization of vulvodynia do not report a higher incidence of childhood physical and sexual abuse (Edwards, Mason, Phillips, Norton, & Boyle, 1997).

Sexual Features

It is clear that women with vulvar vestibulitis do differ from women in comparison groups on many different dimensions of sexuality. Women with vulvar vestibulitis report lower sexual arousal than women in comparison groups (Meana et al., 1997; Nunns & Mandal, 1997; Van Lankveld et al., 1996; White & Jantos, 1998), and lower frequency of intercourse (Meana et al., 1997; Nunns & Mandal, 1997). Women with vulvar vestibulitis also report that they refuse their partners sexual advances more often than women in comparison groups (White & Jantos, 1998), and they differ on sexual satisfaction, sexual schema, sexual behavior and sexual depression (Gates & Galask, 2001). Additionally, women have reported distress over their genital pain with intercourse (Van Lankveld et al., 1996). White and Jantos (1998) found that women with vulvar vestibulitis do not differ from women in a comparison group on sexual desire and frequency of orgasm. However, Meana et al. (1997) found a significant difference between groups on both desire and orgasm. In one retrospective study, the majority of women reported decreases since onset of the disorder in sexual interest, sexual desire, sexual arousal, and activity (Jantos & White, 1997).

Although women report pain with intercourse, research findings indicate that these couples infrequently used other forms of sexual intimacy (Gates & Galask, 2001; Reed, Haefner, Punch, Roth, Gorenflo, & Gillespie, 2000). There is not any data on why women would continue to have vaginal intercourse when it causes them pain. Some hypotheses include: pressure from the partner, a desire for intimacy, other forms of sexual activity are undesirable, and cultural influences that dictate that pain during intercourse for women is acceptable (Hallam-Jones, Wylie, Osborne-Cribb, Harrington, & Walters, 2001). In a discussion of women with vulvar cancer, Van de Wiel, Weijmar Schultz, Wouda, and Bouma (1990) questioned whether or not women who experienced pain with vaginal intercourse had intercourse only to please their partner. The authors hypothesized that the disparity between wants and behavior may be due to issues of equity, in that women felt that their partners were giving and supportive and they owed them something in return.

Couple Relationship

According to McCarthy (2002), sexual concerns are "the most commonly cited reason for separation in the first 2 years of marriage" (p. 630).

These concerns may include conflict about sexual relations, infertility problems, an extramarital affair, and sexual dysfunction. Given that sexual concerns are so important to a marriage, examining the marriages of people with sexual difficulties would seem to be a necessary component of investigating the lives of women with vulvar vestibulitis. Schover et al. (1992) found that women reported on the Dyadic Adjustment Scale similar scores to the normed population. However, they also report that during a standardized interview, women with vulvar vestibulitis reported high levels of marital conflict. Van Lankveld et al. (1996) reported that both men and women in their sample reported normal levels of marital satisfaction.

Data on psychological profiles of male partners of women with vulvar vestibulitis have demonstrated that they are not different than a normal population in regards to psychopathology or psychological distress (Van Lankveld et al., 1996). However, this is the only study that has reported any data on the partner's distress or psychological symptoms. As research with the women with vulvar vestibulitis has been somewhat contradictory, it may be that research of partners also needs to be replicated before a clear picture is elucidated.

Further study needs to be done on the marital interactions of couples in this population in order to determine if their marriages differ from marriages in the general population. It may be that standardized assessments do not capture the subtleties of how couples make sense of the influence this syndrome has upon their sexual and marital lives. Qualitative work would provide a window into their lives, and how couples cope and adjust to the disruption of their lives. Additionally, further research may provide how distress in relationships influences the physical manifestation of the disorder.

IMPLICATIONS FOR THERAPY

Women with vulvar vestibulitis may appear for therapy for a variety of reasons. They may appear before they have received any type of diagnosis and could present with a complaint of dyspareunia. Or they may present with other issues, and only after thorough assessment, the therapist learns of dyspareunia. In this section, implications for individual, marital, and/or sex therapy will be considered. Although some interventions suggested are aimed only at the woman with vulvar vestibulitis, because of the impact the syndrome often has on the sexual relationship, it is recommended that if she has a partner that the partner be included in the therapy.

It is important that women reporting dyspareunia be assessed for vulvar vestibulitis. Before a therapist proceeds with treatment for dyspareunia, it is important that they determine if a physiological condition is contributing to the pain, and if there are medical treatments available to go along with any necessary psychological and/or couple treatment. For women who were not experiencing psychological distress when first experiencing dyspareunia, a diagnosis of sexual dysfunction secondary to a physiological condition could be given (White & Jantos, 1998). For some women, psychological distress may have exacerbated the manifestation of vulvar vestibulitis, and then a diagnosis of a combination of psychological and physiological effects is appropriate (White & Jantos, 1998).

Because many women have been to several doctors, and through several treatments, they are in need of support. They may feel frustrated with the process, and may have been told by more than one professional that the pain they feel is only in their head (Binik, Bergeron, & Khalife, 2000). Therapy should include reassuring women that their symptoms may not be psychogenic in origin, and psychological distress may be secondary to the pain they are experiencing (White & Jantos, 1998). Women can be encouraged that a combination of medical and psychological treatment may help alleviate the pain they are experiencing. Additionally, therapy may include educating the partner on the biological features of vulvar vestibulitis. Couples should be encouraged to include the partner at the next gynecological examination.

If medical treatment does not alleviate her pain, there is likely to be some grief over the chronicity of the problem and perceived losses. She may have to make some meaning for herself as to what it means to have a chronic disorder (McDaniel, Hepworth, & Doherty 1992). Furthermore, the meaning the couple attributes to her disorder should also be assessed; for example, determining whether either partner attributes the cause to punishment for sexual activities (Binik et al., 2000). Both are losing an activity that they may have enjoyed, and may have viewed sexual intercourse as part of their sexual identity. Additionally, the couple may want children and may be adjusting to losses often associated with infertility. Each of these issues could be addressed in therapy, as the couple struggles to make this part of their identity.

Binik et al. (2000) suggest that vulvar vestibulitis has a biopsychosocial nature, as chronic pain often does. They propose that although vulvar vestibulitis may have a physiological origin, psychological processes can contribute to the worsening of symptoms. As the woman experiences pain with intercourse, her muscles in her vulvar region begin to tense when anticipating touch or friction. This in turn will influence arousal and lubrication, thus increasing the likelihood of further pain. Interventions aimed at teaching women how to relax their vaginal muscles, use a vaginal dilator, and use biofeedback are all useful means of helping women decrease the amount of pain they experience (Binik et al., 2000). As indicated above, women with vulvar vestibulitis may have a higher incidence of depression, somatization, and anxiety. Issues of psychological distress or psychopathology should be assessed, and could be treated in either individual or marital therapy. Coping with stress either resulting from, or contributing to, pain is particularly relevant to this population (Binik et al., 2000).

Several behavioral suggestions have been made by the National Association of Vulvodynia (2002) that may help minimize irritation. These include behaviors such as wearing only cotton underwear, loose pants or skirts, no pantyhose, minimizing contact with chemicals (e.g., some laundry detergents, chlorine), using a lubricant during intercourse, and restricting bicycling or horseback riding. Often women only need to be made aware of these behavioral changes, but some may need some coaching on complying with these suggestions. For a woman who does not make behavioral changes, the therapist should assess why. If she does state that she wants to minimize irritation but does not comply with medical advice, the therapist can help explore possible reasons for the contradiction. For example, maybe she feels hopeless about the possibility of changing her circumstances, in which case the therapist can focus on improving her sense of agency in a situation that appears to be out of her control (McDaniel et al., 1992).

If a couple continues to have intercourse when she reports pain with intercourse, a therapist could also help couples explore reasons they continue to have intercourse if she is in pain. Possibly, she does not feel the pain until after intercourse and is accepting of moments of pain for moments of pleasure. But if intercourse is miserable for her, the couple should explore why she is willing to continue and why her partner is willing to participate. Is she being honest with her partner about the level of pain that she is enduring? If not, what in their relationship is preventing her being forthcoming with this important communication? If the couple is searching for means of connecting sexually, they may not recognize that there are other means of sexual connection besides vaginal intercourse. The couple together could explore the origins of these beliefs, such as what they have learned from the culture around them about what is "the right way of doing it." Through couple therapy, a couple could explore what their goals of sexual intimacy are and develop means for achieving those goals in less painful ways.

CONCLUSION

Because vulvar vestibulitis syndrome is related to problematic sexual experiences, it is important that therapists who work with couples be aware of this disorder. In some cases, the therapist may be the first professional to hear about the vulvar pain, and therefore needs to refer the woman to a gynecologist for further assessment. There are many behavioral and medical interventions available to women with vulvar vestibulitis. Therefore, it is important that therapists recognize the physiological component to this disorder. Additionally, for some women and couples, losses may accompany this disorder. The therapist can help attend these losses and help women and couples develop coping strategies to the potential changes in their sexual lives. Issues of sexual identity and body image may also need to be addressed, as the woman develops a sexual identity that incorporates issues of illness. The road to diagnosis can often be a painful experience for women, but it is important that women are provided with hope that there is help available for decreasing pain and developing new strategies of living with this disorder.

REFERENCES

Bergeron, S., Binik, Y. M., Khalife, S., Meana, M., Berkley, K. J., & Pagidas, K. (1997a). The treatment of vulvar vestibulitis syndrome: Towards a multimodal approach. *Sexual and Marital Therapy, 12*(4), 305-311.

Bergeron, S., Binik, Y. M., Khalife, S., & Pagidas, K. (1997b). Vulvar vestibulitis syndrome: A critical review. *The Clinical Journal of Pain, 13*, 27-42.

Binik Y. M., Bergeron, S., & Khalife, S. (2000). Dyspareunia. In S. R. Leiblum, & R. C. Rosen (Eds.), *Principles and practice of sex therapy* (3rd edition) (pp. 154-180). New York: Guilford.

Byth, J. L. (1998). Understanding vulvodynia. *Australian Journal of Dermatology, 39*, 139-150.

Edwards, L., Mason, M., Phillips, M., Norton, J., & Boyle, M. (1997). *The Journal of Reproductive Medicine, 42*(3), 135-139.

Friedrich, E. G. (1987). Vulvar vestibulitis syndrome. *Journal of Reproductive Medicine, 32*(2), 110-114.

Gates, E. A., & Galask, R. P. (2001). Psychological and sexual functioning in women with vulvar vestibulitis. *Journal of Psychosomatic Obstetrics & Gynecology, 22*(4), 221-228.

98   *FEMINIST PERSPECTIVES IN MEDICAL FAMILY THERAPY*

ular vestibulitis: Prevalence and historic features in a general gynecologic practice population. *American Journal of Obstetrics and Gynecology, 164*(6), 1609-1616.

Hallam-Jones, R., Wylie, K. R., Osborne-Cribb, J., Harrington, C., & Walters, S. (2001). Sexual difficulties within a group of patients with vulvodynia. *Sexual and Relationship Therapy, 16*(2), 113-126.

Jantos, M., & White, G. (1997). The vestibulitis syndrome: Medical and psychosexual assessment of a cohort of patients. *The Journal of Reproductive Medicine, 42*(3), 145-152.

McCarthy, B. W. (2002). Sexuality, sexual dysfunction, and couple therapy. In A. S. Gurman & Jacobson, N. S. (Eds.), *Clinical handbook of couple therapy* (3rd ed.) (pp. 629-652). New York: Guilford.

McDaniel, S. H., Hepworth, J., & Doherty, W. J. (1992). *Medical family therapy: A biopsychosocial approach to families with health problems.* New York: Basic Books.

Meana, M., Binik, Y. M., Khalife, S., & Cohen, D. R. (1997). Biopsychosocial profile of women with dyspareunia. *Obstetrics and Gynecology, 90*(4), 583-589.

National Association of Vulvodynia. (2002). Author: http://www.nva.org/

Nunns, D., & Mandal, D. (1997). Psychological and psychosexual aspects of vulvar vestibulitis. *Genitourinary Medicine, 73*, 541-544.

O'Hare, P. M., & Sherertz, E. F. (2000). Vulvodynia: A dermatologist's perspective with emphasis on an irritant contact dermatitis component. *Journal of Women's Health and Gender-Based Medicine, 9*(5), 565-569.

Reed, B. D., Haefner, H. K., Punch, M. R., Roth, R. S., Gorenflo, D. W., & Gillespie, B. W. (2000). Psychosocial and sexual functioning in women with vulvodynia and chronic pelvic pain: A comparative evaluation. *Journal of Reproductive Medicine, 45*(8), 624-632.

Reid, R., Omoto, K. H., Precop, S. L., Berman, N. R., Rutledge, L. H., Dean, S. M., & Pleatman, M. (1995). Flashlamp-excited dye laser therapy of idiopathic vulvodynia is safe and efficacious. *American Journal of Obstetrics and Gynecology, 172*(6), 1684-1701.

Schover, L. R., Youngs, D. D., & Cannata, R. (1992). Psychosexual aspects of the evaluation and management of vulvar vestibulitis. *American Journal of Obstetrics and Gynecology, 167*(3), 630-636.

Van de Wiel, H. B. M., Weijmar Schultz, W. C. M., Wouda, J., & Bouma, J. (1990). Sexual functioning of partners of gynecological oncology patients: A pilot study on involvement, support, sexuality, and relationship. *Sexual and Marital Therapy, 5*(2), 123-130.

Van Lankveld, J. J. D. M., Weijenborg, P. M., & Ter Kuile, M. M. (1996). Psychologic profiles of and sexual function in women with vulvar vestibulitis and their partners. *Obstetrics and Gynecology, 88*(1), 65-70.

Weinstein, K. (1988). *Living with endometriosis: How to cope with the physical and emotional challenges.* New York: Addison Wesley.

White, G., & Jantos, M. (1998). Sexual behavior changes with vulvar vestibulitis syndrome. *Journal of Reproductive Medicine, 43*(9), 783-789.

Gender Roles and the Family Life Cycle: The Case of Women with Cancer

Larra Petersen
Theresa Kruczek
Angela Shaffner

SUMMARY. A woman's diagnosis of cancer affects the family system by requiring families to accommodate new daily routines, redistribute roles, develop a new sense of normalcy, and anticipate future changes in family functioning. Gender-role socialization influences the family's ability to adapt to the myriad of changes necessary during the woman's treatment and recovery from cancer. This article integrates knowledge of gender-role socialization within the context of family systems principles and family life cycle stages in order to provide a framework for working with female cancer patients and their families. A case application exemplifying the unique struggle of women diagnosed within the context of the family life cycle is provided. *[Article copies available for a fee from The Haworth Document Delivery Service: 1-800-HAWORTH. E-mail address: <docdelivery@haworthpress.com> Website: <http://www.HaworthPress.com> © 2003 by The Haworth Press, Inc. All rights reserved.]*

Larra Petersen, MA, is currently completing her doctoral studies in Counseling Psychology at Ball State University in Muncie, Indiana. She works at the Cancer Center at Ball Memorial Hospital with patients and families adjusting to cancer (E-mail: larra petersen@juno.com).

Theresa Kruczek, PhD, is Assistant Professor, Counseling Psychology Program, Ball State University.

Angela Shaffner, MA, is a doctoral student in Ball State's Counseling Psychology program.

[Haworth co-indexing entry note]: "Gender Roles and the Family Life Cycle: The Case of Women with Cancer." Petersen, Larra, Theresa Kruczek, and Angela Shaffner. Co-published simultaneously in *Journal of Feminist Family Therapy* (The Haworth Press, Inc.) Vol. 15, No. 2/3, 2003, pp. 99-119; and: *Feminist Perspectives in Medical Family Therapy* (ed: Anne M. Prouty Lyness) The Haworth Press, Inc., 2003, pp. 99-119. Single or multiple copies of this article are available for a fee from The Haworth Document Delivery Service [1-800-HAWORTH, 9:00 a.m. - 5:00 p.m. (EST). E-mail address: docdelivery@haworthpress.com].

KEYWORDS. Feminist family therapy, gender roles, family life cycle, cancer

Women have a one in three lifetime risk of developing cancer (Kayser, Sormanti, & Strainchamps, 1999). Lung, breast, and colorectal cancers account for the highest cancer death rates among women in North America (American Cancer Society, 2003). It is estimated that in 2003 over 211,000 new cases of breast cancer alone will be diagnosed in women (American Cancer Society, 2003). The clinical course of cancer is unique from other illnesses, and influences the situational stressors patients face (Nicholas & Veach, 2000). The disease process begins like other illnesses with initial symptoms, followed by a medical workup and diagnosis. Treatment decisions are then based on the stage of the cancer and can be especially difficult when the disease is in an advanced stage. Unlike many other diseases, often there is not one clearly best treatment option. Women must consider their unique personal, situational, and life stage variables within the context of quality of life versus quantity of life. Treatment may last weeks or months and the side effects from treatment can be debilitating. When treatment has been "effective" the cancer patient undergoes a period of rehabilitation and remission. In these cases, women may experience cancer as a chronic illness, with long-term disabilities. For others, recurrence and further treatment will occur, and this cycle may repeat several times. If the disease continues to progress, the focus shifts to palliative care and quality rather than quantity of life (Nicholas & Veach, 2000).

Cancer patients in general struggle with issues of remission, relapse, deterioration, long-term survival and fear/uncertainty about recurrence (Lederberg, 1998). Female cancer patients not only have to deal with the general issues related to cancer, but also gender-specific issues. Women must make treatment decisions that affect their body image (e.g., lumpectomy vs. mastectomy) and future reproductive options. Women in remission may also struggle with quality of life issues specifically related to their cancer treatment such as lymphedema, following breast cancer surgery (Radina & Armer, 2001). While women with cancer face the aforementioned challenges, they also encounter a myriad of social and environmental influences on their adaptation to the illness. Few studies have investigated the effect of a woman's cancer within the context of one of the most significant sources of social influence, her family. The literature that is available highlights the reciprocal nature of the effect of cancer on the overall functioning of the woman and her family.

The diagnosis of cancer requires significant adaptability for a woman because she must carry on family and life responsibilities while also attending to her own illness. Likewise, cancer limits a woman's personal and interpersonal functioning in ways that require the family system to accommodate new daily routines, redistribute roles, develop a new sense of normalcy, offer her emotional support and anticipate future changes in family functioning (Lewis & Hammond, 1992). The family's ability to adapt to these changes significantly affects her treatment and recovery process. The woman with cancer can focus more on self-care when her family provides her with greater instrumental and emotional support (Jacobs et al., 1998; Veach, Nicholas, & Barton, 2002). The following case example is provided to illustrate the reciprocal nature of the effect of cancer on one woman and her family.

CASE STUDY

"Patricia" is a 42-year-old, divorced, Caucasian female diagnosed with stage IV breast cancer. During her initial diagnosis, she had surgery to remove a large tumor. Following this surgery, "things got back to normal" for a while and she returned to work. However, a few months later she began experiencing soreness in her back which led to the identification of her recurrence of cancer. She reported feeling shocked and stressed, and she felt the recurrence was more difficult to cope with than the initial diagnosis. Patricia faced many disconcerting questions. First and foremost, she questioned who would care for her 11-year-old son, Jason, while she had her radiation treatments. During Patricia's initial diagnosis and treatment, her ex-mother-in-law helped with his care. However, her former mother-in-law's recent diagnosis with colon cancer prevented her from currently providing significant support. Furthermore, Patricia divorced her first husband, Jason's father, ten years previously when Jason was an infant. Jason rarely saw his father, even though they lived in the same community. Patricia attributed this lack of contact to the father's girlfriend's jealous feelings and lack of commitment to Jason's care. However, Patricia was engaged to Charles, who had a good relationship with Jason. Jason referred to Charles as "Dad" and indicated that he enjoyed their time together. Patricia and Charles planned on marrying in the near future, although the date was tentative due to uncertainty about her course of treatment. Patricia described Charles as supportive of her and her struggles with cancer. In addition to the support from Charles, Patricia's mother also provided some instrumental support, but little emotional support. Specifically, she helped Patricia with cooking and housework. Although Patricia required continued assistance and support, she hoped to return to work soon, since she identified experiencing financial stress and pressure to provide for her family.

Patricia's radiation oncologist referred her to a psychotherapist for evaluation of her psychosocial adjustment to her illness. The counselor met with her son as well, since Patricia was concerned about his adjustment to her illness. Her concerns about him arose after the school counselor called to inform her that Jason was frequently tearful at school. Patricia indicated he never displayed these feelings at home. Through counseling it became clear that Patricia's illness was disruptive to her family and life roles and that she was having difficulty adapting to her illness. In particular, Patricia emphasized her disappointment with the lack of informational support that she received from her medical providers regarding her prognosis and the potential effect of that prognosis on her family plans. As her prognosis was poor, Patricia was forced to consider options for her son after her death. She primarily considered two options for him: living with a maternal aunt and uncle, or moving into his dad's home.

In addition to concerns about her death, she identified that the family structure was shifting as Jason had begun to adopt a caretaking role. Specifically, he had begun making dinner and caring for his mother when she was fatigued and weak. She recognized this occurrence as a breached generational boundary, but in the face of limited resources was uncertain how to decrease the burden on her son. In addition, Jason was struggling with the normative developmental challenges of establishing his identity. For example, as he began adopting communal roles not typically expected from a child his age, he was at risk for confusion about healthy roles in adult-adult relationships. A concern was that this childhood pattern of relating could lead to dependency in his adult intimate relationships.

Treatment involved collaborating with the client and utilizing various strategies for maintaining healthy expression of both focus on self (agency) and others (communion) for all members. Counseling was used to provide a forum for discussion on the agentic and communal needs for Patricia and her family. For instance, Patricia was encouraged to demonstrate agency in seeking out informational support from her medical providers. She also was encouraged to exercise agency in two other areas: making treatment decisions based on her quality and quantity of life concerns and identifying her preference for who would care for Jason after her death.

Through this process Patricia identified that her fiancé, Charles, provided the majority of her emotional support and care for Jason. However, she identified problems with her social network and communion needs. Therefore, she was encouraged to increase communion by expanding her emotional resource base and developing a stronger support network among her friends and spiritual community. She also used counseling to devise strategies to communicate more frequently and effectively with her ex-husband and extended family in order to meet Jason's needs for relational functioning, given the impending loss of his mother. Ultimately, the intervention strategies were designed to address the effect of gender-role issues on family functioning for Patricia when coping with her cancer.

GENDER-ROLE SOCIALIZATION AND CANCER

This case highlights many of the unique issues faced by women with cancer, particularly the struggle to balance agency and communion. Bakan (1966) postulated two fundamental modalities of human existence related to masculinity and femininity: agency and communion. Agency refers to being independent, active, competitive, decisive, committed (to goals), self-confident, and self-assured. Communion includes being emotional, gentle, helpful, kind, warm, aware (of feelings), and sympathetic (Spence, Helmreich, & Holahan, 1979). Early theorists investigating agency and communion viewed agentic traits as more positive when expressed in males and communal traits more positive when expressed by females (Buss, 1990; Helgeson, 1993; McCreary & Korabic, 1994; Spence et al., 1979). Although current research acknowledges the positive nature of the agency and communion constructs, it also identifies the undesirable or unmitigated components of the traits and the disproportionate effect of these traits on men and women, particularly in the areas of interpersonal relationships and psychological well-being (Helgeson, 1994). Specifically, Spence and colleagues (1979) identify unmitigated agency, which is more common in males, as being the most socially undesirable aspect of agency. Helgeson and Fritz (2000) note that unmitigated agency and agency have the commonality of focus on self but the unmitigated construct includes the focus on the self to the exclusion of others. In contrast, unmitigated communion, which is more commonly identified among women, involves two features of concern in relation to interpersonal functioning: over-involvement and self-neglect (Helgeson, 1994; Fritz & Helgeson, 1998). Consistent with gender-role theory, individuals possessing the unmitigated traits have more difficulty adjusting to cancer (Helgeson & Lepore, 1997; Piro et al., 2001). While gender socialization is not as rigid today as in previous generations, studies show that socialization continues to shape gender-role behaviors (Jacklin, 1989).

Gender-role socialization is the primary process contributing to an imbalance in household responsibilities within couples and families (Freidan, 1997). Traditionally, women have carried a disproportionate burden with regard to household tasks. The imbalance becomes more evident and problematic in the case of cancer. Specifically, the diagnosis of a woman's cancer often requires shifts in family roles with regard to instrumental behaviors, such as household chores and childcare. The family's ability to meet the instrumental and emotional needs of a woman with cancer is, in part, influenced by gender-role socialization. Further, many women try to maintain all pre-cancer tasks and resist asking for help in an attempt to avoid further change and perceived additional stress to the family system (Vess, Moreland, & Schwebel, 1985). Reallocation of role responsibility is easier in family systems demonstrating gender role flexibility. Essentially in healthy families, when the female cancer patient asks for assistance, members respond by redistributing tasks among other capable members, regardless of gender.

FAMILY SYSTEMS AND THE FAMILY LIFE CYCLE

The effect of gender-role socialization on the healthy adjustment of women and their families to the diagnosis and treatment of cancer must be understood within the context of family systems theory and the family life cycle. Family systems theory, the application of general systems theory to family functioning, is the dominant model for investigating the effect of stress on the family system (Jacobs et al., 1998). Family systems theory focuses on the extent to which the family system changes its structure and functions across the life cycle in response to both normative developmental changes and stressors, such as cancer (Goldenberg & Goldenberg, 1998; Nichols & Swartz, 1995; Olson & Lavee, 1989). Carter and McGoldrick's (1989) family life cycle theory suggests the female cancer patient is part of a multigenerational system moving vertically (patterns of relating transmitted across generations) and horizontally (normative development and unpredictable stressors) through the life cycle. The interaction of the vertical and horizontal axes occurs when past patterns guide present crisis appraisal, resource management, and expectation of success or failure (Lederberg, 1998). For example, if a grandparent has suffered greatly from complications to cancer treatment, then the woman with cancer and her family are more likely to react strongly to her diagnosis and treatment of cancer because of their past experience and assumptions about the progression of the illness. Therefore, addressing unique family patterns arising in family systems is important for healthy adjustment in families.

Family Systems and Cancer

Healthy adjustment in families where a woman has cancer depends on the core systems principles of cohesion, adaptability/flexibility, communication, and family roles (Goldenberg & Goldenberg, 1998; Veach et al., 2002), and these principles must be understood within the context of the family lifecycle (Carter & McGoldrick, 1989). First, cohesion refers to the emotional connection family members feel towards one another (Veach et al., 2002). In healthy families, the members remain individuated from but connected to each other. In the case of a woman with cancer, her family would remain involved in her care while continuing obligatory life tasks, such as work or school. In contrast, unhealthy families show patterns where members are enmeshed or disengaged. As Sherman and Simonton (2001) note, it is important to assess and address both enmeshment and disengagement because of their negative effect on cancer adjustment.

Enhancing cohesion in disengaged families with cancer is essential because a cohesive family is better able to adapt to the pressures of the illness by shifting roles, responsibilities, and boundaries over the course of the illness (Sherman & Simonton, 2001). Disengaged family members may show a tendency to move further away from the woman in times of stress or crisis (Sherman & Simonton, 2001). The process of outreach and involvement of the disengaged family members should be gradual. One relatively nonthreatening way to involve a disengaged family member of a woman with cancer is to have them take her to initial medical appointments. This low level of involvement begins building bridges between the family and the disengaged member while paving the way for increased involvement and support as her treatment progresses.

Likewise, enhancing differentiation is important in enmeshed families in order to avoid the family becoming engulfed by efforts to accommodate the illness (Rolland, 1989; Sherman & Simonton, 2001; Veach et al., 2002). The diagnosis and treatment of cancer eclipses all else in the family when the woman becomes the central component of family functioning. Individual members become focused almost exclusively on the emotional and physical needs of the woman with cancer (Sherman & Simonton, 2001). Conversely, the unspoken rules of an enmeshed family can dictate subjugation of the woman's needs in an attempt to maintain all pre-illness routines. When the woman subjugates her cancer treatment needs in order to maintain a pre-illness façade there is a collective denial of the illness. Ultimately, these families should be encouraged to maintain a balanced perspective which highlights non-illness interests, strengths and resources of the female cancer patient as well as other family members while meeting the instrumental and emotional needs of the woman with cancer. Healthy differentiation is particularly important in coping with cancer in order to avoid caregiver burnout and minimize the risk of suppressing the woman's role as a contributing member of the family (Rolland, 1989; Veach et al., 2002).

The family's adaptability in response to the illness is also important for healthy adjustment to a woman's cancer diagnosis and treatment. Jacobs and colleagues (1998) describe a healthy family as cohesive, integrated, and self-stabilizing. Healthy families demonstrate a resilient capacity to change, manifest by learning new ways of solving problems or modifying roles in response to stressors such as cancer. Patterson (1988) proposed the Family Adjustment and Adaptation Response (FAAR) Model to describe healthy adaptation to unexpected stress, such as a diagnosis with cancer. The diagnosis and subsequent treatment causes a crisis until the family develops new resources or coping strategies to deal with the stress of the illness. In particular, reducing the number or stressors addressed by the family and reframing the meaning of the stressors for the family can facilitate healthy adaptation to her cancer.

Typical stressors for women with cancer often involve quality of life issues resulting from undergoing adjuvant therapies (chemotherapy and radiation therapy) and secondary effects from cancer (e.g., lymphedema, or fluid buildup in tissues surrounding removed lymph nodes, typical in breast cancer survivors). Women coping with cancer also often struggle with balancing their increased dependence on others with the sense of identity they historically have gained from independent responsibility for family matters (Allen & Hawkins, 1999). In particular, family members may foster unhealthy adaptation and unintentionally hinder the woman's functional recovery by encouraging her to remain physically inactive during the adjuvant treatment process (Bolger et al., 1996).

Healthy adaptation for these women and their families will involve making adjustments to the tasks the woman is able to successfully complete, rather than encouraging her to avoid them (Radina & Armer, 2001).

For example, when a woman experiences lymphedema, she will not be able to lift more than 10 pounds, make repetitive movements, or have full mobility in the affected arm. Therefore, family members need to be patient with the increased time it takes her to complete tasks or she may need facilitative devices to perform tasks. However, her ability to successfully complete the tasks in a modified fashion not only enhances her sense of agency, but also enables her to remain a valuable resource within the family. In some cases, the woman will need to rely on family members or even outside agencies for assistance with household tasks and treatment. When this happens, healthy adaptation can be facilitated by clear communication about both the logistics of realigned responsibilities and the emotional effect of these changes on all family members (Bolger et al., 1996).

Furthermore, it is important to foster healthy communication in families with cancer as poor communication adversely affects adjustment, treatment adherence, and potentially, survivability (Gotcher, 1993; Sherman & Simonton, 2001). While successful adjustment to cancer requires constructive discussions, often the illness brings silence to family communications. Specifically, women with cancer report being dissatisfied with the quality and quantity of communication that occurs in the family about their illness. This dissatisfaction frequently results from women having difficulty communicating about their illness and their corresponding emotional distress because they do not want to "burden" their family (Gotcher, 1993). Likewise, the family avoids initiating discussions about the illness or the woman's experience for fear of "saying the wrong thing" or upsetting her further (Gotcher, 1993; Veach et al., 2002). Ultimately, the family's difficulties communicating about the distress caused by cancer may, in part, be a function of traditional gender roles. Specifically, women traditionally serve a more communal role in families than men, and deviation from these traditional roles creates imbalance and uncertainty for both parties (Rolland, 1989).

Healthy families also use clear communication (congruence between verbal messages and metacommunication) to establish roles and boundaries between subsystems and generations (Barnhill, 1979; Nichols & Minuchin, 1999). Boundaries define and protect the integrity of these subsystems and lay the foundation for identified family roles (Vetere, 2001). Healthy families contain members who balance agency and communion, and who can demonstrate gender role flexibility in times of stress (Helgeson, 1993; 1994). Role reciprocity allows both men and women to be more central in family functioning (communion) while continuing to maintain a focus on self and personal needs (agency). In contrast, unhealthy families demonstrate rigidity in their roles characteristic of the unmitigated extremes. For example, an unmitigated agentic partner may be unable to subsume family responsibilities because of his extreme focus on himself and his personal goals. Furthermore, an unmitigated communion woman is unable to allow others to assist her with self-care, child-care, and household responsibilities because of the over-involvement with others and self-neglect characteristic of women with this trait. In contrast to those families possessing unmitigated traits, healthy families with balanced gender roles react by adjusting family roles based on appropriate shifts in responsibility, between and within generations in various life cycle stages (Carter & McGoldrick, 1989).

Family Life Cycle and Cancer

Since women traditionally have been identified as central to the functioning of the family system and life cycle, their diagnosis with cancer places more stress on the family system and makes the family more vulnerable to disruption of normal family development (McGoldrick, 1989). Specifically, when the woman is not available to carry the burden of the family's emotional needs, due to cancer, the family may fail to accomplish the emotional processes necessary for successful transitions between life cycle or developmental stages. Successful progression through the family life cycle depends on many illness and family variables. Illness variables may include type or site of cancer, stage of cancer, course of treatment (i.e., radiation and chemotherapy), and outcome of treatment (Veach et al., 2002). The family variables of cohesion, adaptability/flexibility, communication, and family roles, discussed earlier, vary in significance depending on the life cycle stage of the family.

As the family life cycle is a model based on chronological time, it is important to note the multigenerational and parallel nature of the stages. Specifically, at a given point in time there could be three women in the multigenerational system at three different lifecycle stages coping with a woman's diagnosis of cancer. For example, the youngest woman might be in the first stage, leaving home, while her mother is in the fifth stage, launching children, and her grandmother in the final stage, families later in life. The core developmental issues at each life cycle stage will be reviewed within the context of a woman with cancer at that stage, followed by a discussion of the effect of cancer on the family at that stage. Also, the role of agency and communion will be described and implications for treatment provided at each stage.

Stage one: Leaving home. In the first stage the emphasis is on the identity processes of separation and individuation (Haley, 1997). Essentially, the young woman is working to successfully establish a balance between continuity and innovation, develop intimate peer relationships, and establish her emotional and financial independence (Carter & McGoldrick, 1999). Women at this stage strive to develop a balance between agency or focus-on-self and communion or a sense of connectedness. Ultimately, these processes are centrifugal, such that they propel the young woman away from her family of origin while encouraging her to remain involved in social networks.

The diagnosis of cancer for a young, single woman affects her accomplishment of these life cycle tasks in three key ways. First, the diagnosis disrupts the process of establishing herself in work and intimate relationships. The centripetal force of the diagnosis often pulls the woman back into her family of origin, which is counter to the normative developmental process of separation and individuation. The more debilitating her treatment and course of illness, the more likely she will experience difficulty mastering the tasks of innovation and continuity. Second, this pull back into the family of origin may impede her successful formation of intimate peer relationships, particularly partner relationships. Finally, the young woman with cancer may be particularly vulnerable to the issues of body image and sexuality that can accompany cancer, as identity consolidation is a normative developmental task (Veach et al., 2002).

In addition, the young woman's return to her family of origin can cause disruption in other members' movement through the life cycle stages. For example, her parents' focus on her illness and recovery may interfere with their preparing her younger siblings to leave home. Her stage five parents may also invest more energy in caring for their daughter with cancer than their normative developmental task of rekindling their intimate partner bond. Finally, her return to her family of origin and reliance on them for illness care may delay her stage five mother's individuation from the family and subsequent pursuit of nonfamily interest areas.

In working with the young woman with cancer and her family, it is important to clarify the course of treatment and prognosis. Early identification of possible outcomes can help the young woman realistically appraise her expected level of independence. In cases where long-term survivability is limited, the young woman can work to establish independence within the parameters of the course of the illness. However, in cases where the prognosis is good, she can conceptualize the illness as a temporary setback in her progression through this stage.

Regardless, she should be encouraged to seek out and maintain peer relationships in order to foster developmentally appropriate emotional independence from her family of origin. These young women may grapple with accepting their post cancer appearance and sexuality, particularly with reproductive and breast cancers, as a result of feeling at odds with culturally accepted ideals. Given that identity development is part of the normative process for these young women, it is important to help them establish a healthy sense of self and an acceptance of their bodies (Veach et al., 2002).

Stage two: Joining of families through marriage. The second stage, joining of families, begins with the courtship of a new couple (Carter & McGoldrick, 1989). At this time, the couple has an idealized image of one another and they often overlook the difficulties of merging their two family systems. The new family system requires realignment of extended families and merging of finances, emotions, power, and activities (Carter & McGoldrick, 1989). Both partners in the couple negotiate a healthy balance of maintaining independence (agency) achieved at stage one with continued involvement in original and newly established social networks (communion).

When a woman is diagnosed with cancer at this stage, however, there is often an imbalance of agency and communion. For example, she may, at least temporarily, become more physically and emotionally dependent on her partner. Lewis and Hammond (1992) note that the healthy partner often reports feeling inadequate and unprepared to help the woman with cancer cope with the emotional and physical demands accompanying her cancer and its treatment. The partner often feels insecure assuming these roles in the newly emerging family system. The authors also identify that when the woman's partner had difficulty managing their own emotional reactions, making decisions, adjusting to new life responsibilities, or providing emotional support, depression increases for both the woman and partner. This depression creates greater dissatisfaction with the relationship for both. In turn, the dissatisfaction causes the woman to pull away from the newly forming relationship and move toward her family of origin, essentially resulting in a breached generational boundary. When this process occurs, the cancer serves to delay the merging of the new couple (Veach et al., 2002). When women experience greater mutuality and communion in the couple relationship, with regard to emotional experience and role adjustment, they report decreased depression and increased quality of life, self-care, and illness adjustment (Lewis & Hammond, 1992). Therefore, treatment should involve fostering mutuality and clear communication as key elements for healthy adjustment at this stage. Successful couples will maintain their connection and commitment to their relationship while also accessing extended family members for emotional and instrumental aid. Finally, mutual decisions about how to involve their families of origin in care and support of the female cancer patient will maintain the newly forming couple dyad while providing the additional resources the couple may need to cope with the illness (Patterson, 1988).

Stage three: Families with young children. In the third stage, families with young children, the focus is on acceptance of new members into the system (Carter & McGoldrick, 1989). New parents must adjust the couple dyad to accommodate their role as parents as well as partners (Aponte & VanDeusen, 1981). The new parents must make space for the child in the system and renegotiate their own roles with regard to child-rearing, financial, and household tasks (Carter & McGoldrick, 1999). Typically, the changes required at this stage "combine to produce a strong shift of power . . . back toward the traditional arrangement of breadwinner dad and domestic mom" (Carter & McGoldrick, 1999, p. 254). The woman finds herself pushed to more of a communal focus than earlier stages. In contrast, the couple relationship may become more imbalanced with the partner maintaining or moving towards a more agentic focus. Successful negotiation of the increased tasks at this stage requires that new parents integrate an awareness of traditional gender roles and power imbalances often inherent in parenting young children, with the continued need for a healthy balance of agency and communion for both parents.

Little is known about the effect of cancer on the family at this time. However, the available research suggests cancer has a significant influence on the family system when the patient is a woman with young children (Lewis & Hammond, 1992). Women often are already experiencing considerable role strain within the family system at this stage. When they are diagnosed with cancer, these women experience substantial conflict between managing their family responsibilities and self-care needs, especially when other members in the system are unable or unwilling to assume increased responsibility (Kayser et al., 1999). When investigating the effect of cancer on families at this stage, Lewis and Hammond (1992) found that these mothers often report lower marital adjustment that adversely affects the overall functioning of the entire household.

Furthermore, children (ages 6-10) in the family struggle with their mother's diagnosis as evidenced by their reported fear about the integrity of the family and what might happen to them, especially if the cancer were to recur. These younger children and their older counterparts (ages 10-13) experienced sadness, fear, loneliness, worry, and occasional anger that interfered with their overall individual, social, and family functioning. Additionally, the older children's negative emotional experience appeared to adversely affect their self-esteem. Finally, the older children's social functioning was affected because they were often expected to assume new roles with increased responsibilities in order to offset disruptions to household functioning. Successful adjustment to a diagnosis of cancer at this stage involves addressing the role strain created when the woman is unable to meet both her family responsibilities and self-care needs.

Given the significant demands of parenting at this stage, it is particularly important in treatment to address the parent's role expectations within the context of gender-role socialization. Specifically, couples who demonstrate gender role flexibility will more successfully cope with the role strain created by the woman's cancer. In addition to role shifts within the couple dyad, the children can be involved in accepting developmentally appropriate increased responsibilities within the family. In order to maintain healthy development of the children, it is imperative they are not overburdened and they are encouraged to maintain normative social interaction.

Treatment with children whose mothers have cancer may need to emphasize cognitive understanding of the illness and coping with the negative emotional experiences that accompany their mother's illness. Mastery of their negative emotions can help foster healthy esteem. These children's adjustment can be further enhanced by clear communication between the couple dyad focusing on maintenance of clear generational boundaries with the children and extended family. When illness characteristics suggest the likelihood of untimely death, it is important for parents to prepare the children for impending changes in the family and to identify ways for the woman's extended family to remain involved in the children's life so they do not experience multiple losses as a result of their mother's death. Also, when the woman's death is imminent, it is important for the partners to discuss her wishes in regard to advanced directives.

Stage four: Families with adolescents. During stage four, families with adolescents, the system is working toward increasing the flexibility of family boundaries to encourage the teenager's increased agency and independence (Carter & McGoldrick, 1989). Parent-child relationships must shift to allow the teenager to "move in and out of the system." In addition, the parents begin to shift their communal focus from the children back to the couple (Carter & McGoldrick, 1989). Establishing a balance of agency and communion among all family members is an essential developmental task at this stage. In particular, the mother and adolescent children shift to identify and incorporate more agentic foci within the context of family functioning.

The woman with cancer at this stage may struggle with balancing the normative shifts in agency and communion while managing the increased demands of her medical care. For women working outside the home, cancer can affect their long-term career goals. Promoting agency around career issues will facilitate long-term adjustment for these women and maintain the sense of increased agency that is normative at this stage. For homemakers, cancer can interfere with the normative process of increasing non-childrearing interests and pursuits. While the woman with cancer at this stage will likely struggle with balancing agency and communion, the greater risk to the family system as a whole is breached generational boundaries within the family of procreation (Veach et al., 2002).

The centripetal pull of the cancer diagnosis and treatment not only influences the mother's focus away from her own increased agency, but may also pull her adolescent daughter(s) back into the system to fill both the instrumental and emotional void that can be created by their mother's illness. This process is contrary to the teen's normative centrifugal shift away from the family and toward increased agency. Older adolescent daughters may be especially vulnerable to this role strain when there are younger children in the family. Parents in these families may feel pressured to increase the daughter's responsibilities and restrict their boundaries, thereby limiting her capacity to move out of the system (Veach et al., 2002). This tendency will be especially strong in families holding traditional gender-role expectations, when these young women will be perceived as an additional resource to fill the void left by their mother. Likewise, the female daughters of women with cancer are at increased risk for incorporating unrealistic ideals for caregiving (unmitigated communion) as part of their identity as a result of the extreme influence on caring for others in their formative years. Male and female adolescents whose mother has cancer often experience esteem difficulties, specifically poor self-worth, which ultimately places an additional stress on the family system (Lewis & Hammond, 1992).

In counseling, healthy adjustment can be fostered by clarifying generational boundaries and appropriate roles, particularly with regard to adolescent daughters meeting the emotional and instrumental needs previously met by their now ill mother. Although adolescents are developmentally equipped to carry more responsibility with regard to household tasks, they should be encouraged to maintain peer and leisure involvement as much as possible regardless of gender. In order to reduce the adolescent's burden, the couple dyad can identify ways to garner support from extended family members without breaching generational boundaries. Again, communication and role flexibility between partners can serve to strengthen their relationship and enhance family system functioning.

Stage five: Launching children. The fifth stage, launching children, is the longest phase in the lifecycle and can last 20 years or more. This stage requires that families accept many entries into and exits from the family system (Carter & McGoldrick, 1989). At this stage, there is much realignment in the system as children begin to leave home and introduce new, extended family members via their union with another system. The process of realignment often requires new roles, rules, and subsystem boundaries as parents adopt adult-adult relationships with their children (Carter & McGoldrick, 1989; Veach et al., 2002). Due to the many exits at this stage, many mothers experience "the empty nest" syndrome and as a result often venture outside the family system to incorporate new, non-childcare interests and activities into their identity (Lerner, 1998). The continued shift from a family focus to a self-focus contributes to a change in the balance of agency and communion for the woman individually and within the couple dyad. This shift in focus and change in interests often creates tension in the partner relationship and subsequent couple dyad problems (Carter & McGoldrick, 1999). Healthy families use their communication skills to negotiate these role shifts and balance individual and family needs.

A diagnosis with cancer can be especially difficult in the early years of this stage for women whose primary focus has been homemaking. Her diagnosis and treatment with cancer can interfere with her continued shift away from communal family roles, toward her own personal agentic goals. For women with limited non-childcare interests and activities, the cancer may become the focus of her identity and involvement. While all women treated for cancer at this stage can experience difficulty balancing their own needs for self-care and the needs of their elder relatives, women whose primary focus has been the family may have greater difficulty striking this balance.

The diagnosis and treatment of cancer at this stage also interferes with the normative realignment of relationships between the parents and their adult children. As the woman becomes more debilitated, either because of adjuvant therapies or advanced stages of cancer, her grown children are often drawn back into the family of origin. Again daughters of mothers with cancer are more vulnerable to this pull and may experience conflict between the developmental push to exit the system and start their own family and the pull to remain a part of their family of origin (Veach et al., 2002). This pull is particularly strong for the daughters of women with cancer who exhibit unmitigated communion traits because of their tendency to return to the family of origin to assume the caregiver role for their ill mothers. When this process occurs, it exacerbates the role strain already experienced by this "sandwich generation" of women, who are working to meet the needs of their family of choice as well as the needs of their family of origin.

At this stage, encouraging the woman with cancer and her partner to utilize the resources within their couple dyad to meet her instrumental and emotional needs during her treatment and recovery will enhance healthy adjustment. She and her partner may have to creatively work together to find ways to provide care for their elder relatives without adding to the female cancer patient's role strain. Women with cancer at this stage who have not yet had significant non-childcare interests and activities should be encouraged to explore aspects of their identity beyond the family and their cancer. Further, when the women at this stage are able to promote their adult-to-adult relationships with their adult children, the two generations develop skills necessary to communicate their personal needs and subsequently devise ways to provide for the needs of all generations. For example, when the cancer patient and her adult children experience role strain, they may need to access resources within other parts of their social networks rather than predominantly relying on family members.

Stage six: Families in later life. The primary developmental task in the final stage, families in later life, involves acceptance of shifting generational roles (Carter & McGoldrick, 1989). This stage is characterized by status changes, such as retirement, and the accompanying lifestyle adjustments. One lifestyle adjustment includes financial strain, especially when there is a serious illness such as cancer. Another adjustment includes the increased amount of time partners spend with each other. Couples that have maintained a strong couple dyad throughout the parenting and launching years are able to retain a sense of agency by maintaining their own functioning in the face of physical decline while allowing and even encouraging their adult children to communally explore new family roles in separate subsystems. In addition, successful adaptation to the shrinking community of friends and relatives is facilitated when the couple dyad is strong. Overall, the focus in the aging couple system returns primarily to a communal or systems focus.

As with many life-threatening illnesses, the risk for cancer increases with age. In particular, one in three women copes with a diagnosis of cancer in later life (American Cancer Society, 2003). Schnoll and Harlow (2001) note that older cancer patients often experience less distress associated with their diagnosis because they have previously achieved many of the common developmental tasks of our society. While illness and death are normative at this stage, the woman with cancer may struggle with limited financial and personal resources to cope with the illness. Most often it is the woman's adult children who care for her during her cancer treatment and recovery. This role reversal can be difficult for both child and parent. In healthy families, the parent and adult child negotiate new boundaries such that the adult child provides support, but does not take over functioning for their ill parent (Veach et al., 2002). This role reversal is particularly difficult in traditional, communal families where the mother is perceived as the primary caregiver and emotional stronghold. In treatment, assisting these families with the typical life tasks of this stage may include having the family engage in a life review, identifying resources outside the family system, and realigning the generational roles to accommodate loss of elders.

CONCLUSION

Cancer affects the family system in a multitude of ways. The woman's diagnosis affects the family by forcing adjustment to new and varied roles, rules, and responsibilities. In order to cope with cancer at any given life stage, the family must fill lost roles, cope with demands of the illness, meet family members' emotional needs, and continue progression through the family life cycle. The preceding discussion highlights ways in which gender-role socialization greatly affects the adjustment of the patient and the response of her family to the changes prompted by the clinical course of cancer. Therefore, clinicians working with families affected by cancer should incorporate knowledge of gender-role socialization within the context of general systems principles and the family life cycle. These constructs have been integrated in this paper in order to provide a framework for working with female cancer patients and their families. However, it remains important to note that only a few of the many possible cancer and family scenarios are presented in the context of this paper. Ultimately, this paper strives to provide a nomothetic perspective to coping with cancer in a family consisting of a couple with children. Since variations likely exist for many patients, clinicians are encouraged to utilize the information presented in an ideographic manner to best meet any individual woman's needs.

REFERENCES

Allen, S. M., & Hawkins, A. J. (1999). Maternal gatekeeping: Mothers' beliefs and behaviors that inhibit greater father involvement in family work. *Journal of Marriage and the Family, 61,* 199-212.

American Cancer Society (2003). Cancer facts and figures. Retrieved on May 22, 2003, from *http://www.cancer.org/downloads/STT/CAFF2003PWSecured.pdf.*

Aponte, H. J., & VanDeusen, J. M. (1981). Structural family therapy. In A. Gurman and D. P. Kniskern (Eds.), *Handbook of family therapy* (pp. 310-360). New York: Brunner/Mazel.

Bakan (1966). *The duality of human existence.* Chicago: Rand McNally.

Barnhill, L. R. (1979). Healthy family systems. *The Family Coordinator, January,* 94-100.

Bolger, N., Foster, M., Vinokur, A.D., & Ng, R. (1996). Close relationships and adjustment to a life crisis: The case of breast cancer. *Journal of Personality and Social Psychology, 70,* 283-294.

Buss, D. M. (1990). Unmitigated agency and unmitigated communion: An analysis of the negative components of masculinity and femininity. *Sex Roles, 22,* 555-568.

Carter, B., & McGoldrick, M. (1989). *The changing family lifecycle: A framework for family therapy (2nd ed.).* Needham Heights, MA: Allyn & Bacon.

Carter, B., & McGoldrick, M. (1999). *The extended family lifecycle: Individual, family, and social perspectives (3rd ed.).* Needham Heights, MA: Allyn & Bacon.

Freidan, B. (1997). *Beyond gender: The new politics of work and family.* Washington, D.C.: The Woodrow Wilson Center.

Fritz, H. L., & Helgeson, V. S. (1998). Distinctions of unmitigated communion from communion: Self-neglect and over-involvement with others. *Journal of Personality and Social Psychology, 75,* 121-140.

Goldenberg, I., & Goldenberg, H. (1996). *Family therapy: An overview.* Pacific Grove, CA: Brooks/Cole.

Gotcher, J. M. (1993). The effects of family communication on psychosocial adjustment of cancer patients. *Journal of Applied Communication Research, 17,* 176-188.

Haley, J. (1987). *Problem-solving therapy (2nd ed.).* San Francisco, CA: Jossey-Bass/Pfeiffer.

Haley, J. (1997). *Leaving home: The therapy of disturbed young people (2nd ed.).* Philadelphia: Brunner/Mazel.

Helgeson, V. S. (1993). Implications of agency and communion for patient and partner adjustment to a first coronary event. *Journal of Personality and Social Psychology, 64,* 807-816.

Helgeson, V. S. (1994). Relation of agency and communion to psychological well-being: Evidence and potential explanations. *Psychological Bulletin, 116*, 412-428.
Helgeson, V. S., & Fritz, H. L. (2000). The implications of unmitigated agency and unmitigated communion for domains of problem behavior. *Journal of Personality, 68*, 1031-1056.
Helgeson, V. S., & Lepore, S. J. (1997). Men's adjustment to prostate cancer: The role of agency and unmitigated agency. *Sex Roles, 37*, 251-267.
Jacklin, C. N. (1989). Female and male: Issues of gender. *American Psychologist, 44*, 127-133.
Jacobs, J., Ostroff, J., & Steinglass, P. (1998). Family therapy: A systems approach to cancer care. In J. Holland (Ed.), *Psycho-oncology* (pp. 994-1003). New York: Oxford University.
Kayser, K., Sormanti, M., & Strainchamps, E. (1999). Women coping with cancer: The influence of relationship factors on psychosocial adjustment. *Psychology of Women Quarterly, 23*, 725-739.
Lederberg, M. S. (1998). The family of the cancer patient. In J. Holland (Ed.), *Psycho-oncology* (pp. 981-993). New York: Oxford University.
Lerner (1998). *The mother dance.* New York, NY: Harper Collins.
Lewis, F. M., & Hammond, M. A. (1992). Psychosocial adjustment of the family to breast cancer: A longitudinal analysis. *Journal of the American Medical Women's Association, 47*, 104-200.
McCreary, D. R., & Korabik, K. (1994). Examining the relationships between the socially desirable and undesirable aspects of agency and communion. *Sex Roles, 31*, 637-651.
McGoldrick, M. (1989). Women and the family lifecycle. In B. Carter & M. McGoldrick (Eds.), *The changing family lifecycle: A framework for family therapy (2nd ed.)* (pp. 31-68). Needham Heights, MA: Allyn & Bacon.
Nicholas, D. R., & Veach, T. A. (2000). The psychosocial assessment of the adult cancer patient. *Professional Psychology: Research and Practice, 31*(2), 206-215.
Nichols, M. P., & Minuchin, S. (1998). Structural family therapy. In J. M. Donovan (Ed.), *Short-term couple therapy* (pp. 124-143). New York: Guilford.
Nichols, M. P., & Schwartz, R. C. (1995). *Family therapy: Concepts and methods (3rd ed.).* Boston: Allyn & Bacon.
Olson, D. H. (1993). Circumplex model of marital and family systems: Assessing family functioning. In F. Walsh (Ed.), *Normal family processes.* New York: Guilford.
Olson, D. H., & Lavee, Y. (1989). Family systems and family stress: A family lifecycle perspective. In K. Kreppner & R. M. Lerner (Eds.), *Family systems and life-span development* (pp. 165-195). Hillsdale, NJ: Lawrence Erlbaum.
Patterson, J. M. (1988). Families experiencing stress: The family adjustment and adaptation response model. *Family Systems Medicine, 5*, 202-237.
Piro, M., Zeldrow, P. B., Knight, S. J., Mytko, J. J., & Gradishar, W. J. (2001). The relationship between agentic and communal personality traits and psychosocial adjustment to breast cancer. *Journal of Clinical Psychology in Medical Settings, 8*, 263-271.
Radina, M. E., & Armer, J. M. (2001). Post-breast cancer lymphedema and the family: A qualitative investigation of families coping with chronic illness. *Journal of Family Nursing, 7*, 281-299.

Rolland, J. (1998). Chronic illness and the family lifecycle. In B. Carter & M. McGoldrick (Eds.), *The changing family lifecycle: A framework for family therapy (2nd ed.)* (pp. 433-456). Needham Heights, MA: Allyn & Bacon.
Schnoll, R. A., & Harlow, L. L. (2001). Using disease-related and demographic variables to form cancer-distress risk groups. *Journal of Behavioral Medicine, 24,* 57-73.
Sherman, A. C., & Simonton, S. (2001). Coping with cancer in the family. *Family Journal: Counseling and Therapy for Couples and Families, 9,* 193-200.
Spence, J. T., Helmrich, R. L., & Holahan, C. K. (1979). Negative and positive component of psychological masculinity and femininity and their relationship to self-reports of neurotic and acting out behaviors. *Journal of Personality and Social Psychology, 37,* 1673-1682.
Veach, T. A., Nicholas, D. R., & Barton, M. A. (2002). *Cancer and the family lifecycle: A practitioner's guide.* Lillington, NC: Edwards Brothers.
Vess, J. D., Moreland, J. R., & Schwebel, A. I. (1985). A follow-up study of role functioning and the psychological environment of families of cancer patients. *Journal of Psychosocial Oncology, 3,* 1-14.
Vetere, A. (2001). Structural family therapy. *Child Psychology and Psychiatry Review, 6,* 133-139.
Vinokur, A. D., Threatt, B. A., Caplan, R. D., & Zimmerman, B. L. (1989). Physical and psychosocial functioning and adjustment to breast cancer: Long-term follow-up of a screening population. *Cancer, 63,* 394-405.

REFLECTIONS

Isolation, Depersonalization and Repeat Trauma: Reflections on Surgery During a Hospital Quarantine

Jane McNamee

Day 1. I arrive at the hospital in Ontario, Canada, with my husband. Precautionary screening measures are in place at the entry to the hospital, and all hospitals in the province. This is to prevent the spread of Severe Acute Respiratory Symptom (SARS), a new corona virus, in hospitals or the community. We go to the screening procedure, a large tent where volunteers ask questions about fever, contact and travel, and squirt

Jane McNamee, MA, is a retired research associate and group therapist who, for 15 years, worked for the Canadian Centre for Studies of Children at Risk, and Chedoke Child and Family Centre, Department of Psychiatry, McMaster University, Hamilton, Ontario.

Address correspondence: to Jane McNamee, 15 Westwind Circle, Guelph, Ont. N1G 4Z4, Canada.

The author gratefully acknowledges the editorial contributions of Alexina Murphy, MDiv, and Jean Turner, PhD.

[Haworth co-indexing entry note]: "Isolation, Depersonalization and Repeat Trauma: Reflections on Surgery During a Hospital Quarantine." McNamee, Jane. Co-published simultaneously in *Journal of Feminist Family Therapy* (The Haworth Press, Inc.) Vol. 15, No. 2/3, 2003, pp. 121-125; and: *Feminist Perspectives in Medical Family Therapy* (ed: Anne M. Prouty Lyness) The Haworth Press. Inc., 2003, pp. 121-125. Single or multiple copies of this article are available for a fee from The Haworth Document Delivery Service [1-800-HAWORTH, 9:00 a.m. - 5:00 p.m. (EST). E-mail address: docdelivery@haworthpress.com].

antibiotic soap onto our hands. We pass the screen and are issued with yellow tags for the current date. We are directed to Admissions, and then to Intake for today's surgery. The Intake ward is empty. We are the only people there. Normally it is buzzing with patients and nurses. Two nurses and an orderly take care of us. They all say it is unusually quiet. We think of those people who have had today's surgery cancelled, especially those awaiting donor transplants whose lives are at risk. My surgery has been cancelled twice previously, and I feel fortunate for my slot today.

Eventually I am wheeled to the pre-op area. My husband is allowed to accompany me. It is the last time I see him for five days. I am taken to the operating room where my hip is to be replaced. Later, when I recover consciousness, I look for my husband. Instead I am greeted by my surgeon and his two male residents. They are very animated, their eyes sparkling, big smiles. They look like they've just accomplished a particularly gruelling triathlon. Only later I realise the triathlon has been on my body, specifically my hip. Excitedly they tell me what complicated surgical procedures the three of them have just achieved for my new hip.

> This involved extensive physical handling, starting with dislocation of the original hip joint before removal. The upper end of the thigh bone was removed, and lower down the bone was cut and rotated to correct the foot alignment. A titanium arm, which had a ball at its upper end, was inserted into the top of the bone marrow cavity. Stainless steel wire was wrapped around the thigh bone twice to preventing splitting under pressure. More bone was reamed out from the upper part of the joint, and a titanium cup (mating with the ball) was inserted and held in place with a long screw. The reamed out bone chips were used to build up the area around the cuts in the thigh bone and held in place with wire mesh.

Then they say, "You won't remember this later." Of course I don't remember the details later, but I do remember the reference to forgetfulness, and it really gets up my 65-year-old feminist nose! I am uncertain as to whether the remark relates to objectification of the aging memory, or is a reference to the effects of anaesthetics. In either instance, their thrill with their surgical achievements unintentionally leaves me feeling as just another challenging "case," and unrecognised as a person who has just undergone huge physical trauma to her body.

Days 2, 3, and 4 are full of narcotics, dressings, and catheters. I drift in and out of sleep. Occasionally I notice people signing a sheet on my door. I wonder why they do this since they haven't made any personal contact with me. It turns out that everybody who comes on the ward has to sign a SARS sheet for each patient, every day, whether they have contact with them or not. This is in case any one of us should develop SARS. The cross referencing for this ward alone, with 19 rooms and 60 plus patients, must be monumental. The nurses (both genders) are stretched beyond their limits. They talk about calls for volunteers to run the SARS screen at the hospital doors. I am aware that I do not want to bother them with my requests–to ask that they pass me something I cannot reach, or pick up things I have dropped on the floor. I miss my husband. On my previous hospital stays he has been able to visit me each day and carry out small tasks which made my life more comfortable: He would get me a drink, brush my hair, hold my hand, rub my feet, tell me about his daily life. Now there is no one to walk beside me on this part of my journey.

Day 5. I wake and feel very teary. I can't seem to be able to stop crying. I've noticed I have trouble passing urine. I feel bruised and engorged in my genital area. In my narcotic dazed state I wonder if I now have testicles. I cannot investigate what's going on "down there" as I may not bend more than ninety degrees to protect my new hip. Although I ask to speak to the ward's female physician, the male surgeon and other nurses arrive to examine my swollen genitalia. I feel like a spectacle as they gaze at what I cannot see. Again, I feel like an unusual "case" to be assessed, rather than a person with feelings to be taken into account. My questions and concerns are downplayed. I'm told, "This is a common occurrence for this type of surgery." I am quite unable to verbalize my feelings of vulnerability, and of violation. I discount my tearfulness to the nurses as "I am just having a bad day." One nurse takes pity on me and asks for permission for my husband to visit me. Permission is given. I telephone him. He goes through the SARS screen and arrives at my bedside. One of the first things I ask him is to get me a mirror so that I can see for myself what has happened to me. I am shocked at the bruising, the swelling, and the bulging purple labia. I didn't expect this.

Later, my daughter telephones. I explain my physical state and emotional confusion to her. As I speak I begin to link back to an earlier trauma when I was 5 years old. I was sexually assaulted on the first day of my first school. Back then, during World War II in rural Sussex, village children aged 5 to 16 years were taught in a one-room school. I was the new curate's daughter and I spoke with a different accent. So I needed to be made aware of the pecking order in the school. During recess, aided and abetted by all the other children gathered in the lavatories, I was violated by the largest boy in the school. I fainted at the pain. When I came round I was locked in a cubicle. I howled with pain and rage at the injustice of it. The teacher who let me out–both liberator and jailor from her remark–said, "We won't tell your mother about this, will we?" Of course my mother discovered when she dressed me next morning. She was angry that I had followed the injunctions of my teacher. My parents never spoke with me about it, then or later. They were of the belief that least said, soonest mended. Even the memory was hidden until I was able to work on it in therapy as an adult. Now, isolated and immobilized in postoperative pain, my body remembers, and my emotions besiege me once again. Yet, even as I remember the earlier assault, I gradually become aware of something else; someone else. I am aware of my grandparents' presence with me in my hospital room, Brenda and Alfred, my paternal grandparents, long since dead. Living close to us, they most certainly would have known of my five-year-old experience. I do not specifically recall their comforting me then, but I do remember them comforting me at other times in my childhood. When I was younger, and had other surgeries, my Granny sat beside my hospital bed. She told me her funny and whimsical stories to make me laugh. When I had trouble sleeping, my Grandpa often sat beside my bed and stroked my hair. I felt comforted and cherished by his presence. They knew great sadness and helpless loss themselves; their only daughter died of an undiagnosed illness in 1921, at age 13.

Now, at this moment, in my SARS-isolated room, they are with me again, comforting me in my physical pain, soothing my feelings of violation. How to explain their presence? Perhaps, because I am alone and have no visitors, time and space have been bridged. In rational terms, their company, when I most need it some sixty years after that childhood trauma, does not make sense. Maybe it is only now that I can fully appreciate their caring and loving support.

Day 6. Physiotherapy and learning to manoeuvre my swollen limbs to the washroom, to a chair, and then back to bed all seem to take up much of my day. There is talk of my going to the rehabilitation program. However, because of SARS, the program has withdrawn its weekend passes. I opt for home as soon as possible but am told this might be delayed for a few days.

Day 7. Quite unexpectedly, I am told my bed is needed and I may be able to go home tomorrow. The timing of my discharge changes from moment to moment . . . possibly this evening; no, this afternoon; how soon can I get someone to fetch me? I say, "As soon as my husband can get here!" I leave a few hours later, glad to have the opportunity to begin to reclaim my personal dignity.

Thanks to SARS I have experienced a very unique hospital stay. While there I gained a limited insight into the stress that an epidemic like the SARS virus can put on a medical system. As a 65-year-old woman I chose to have hip surgery unaware that the involuntary trauma experienced by my five-year-old self would return to me. In retrospect, I wonder if the advantage of the isolation created by SARS meant that I was able to process more quickly what was happening to me. If I had been distracted by cheerful friendly visitors with whom I might have felt uncomfortable sharing my story, the parallels between the past and the present experiences might have been lost to me. My aloneness due to the SARS visitor ban meant I had time for reflection on many aspects of my experience of hip surgery. Of course the primary benefit of the surgery is that I now have the gift of a reconstructed hip, a highly skilled and technical achievement that will increase and prolong my mobility. My isolation has made me aware of the importance of the love and support given to me by my grandparents. Upon reflection, I came to understand their loving presence as a unique expression of the universal spirit of love in my life, an expression of God's love for me. I had not fully realised and honoured my grandparent's lifelong support to me until these recent events in the hospital. Now I am aware that the gifts of love and support they gave to me during my life lie within me. They are gifts I wish to give to my own four grandchildren.

I believe this experience has implications on many levels: First, for people who have experienced previous traumas in their lives, that they should be aware that some extensive and physically manipulative surgeries may trigger memories of past experiences. Second, for therapists to work with them ahead of time to activate healing memories to offset the possible effects of surgery and hospitalization, especially in circumstances such as those generated by the isolating effects of SARS or other epidemics. Third, the importance of connection to significant others by phone, through memories, by taking into the hospital any meaningful small object that puts the person in touch with those who care, or cared, for them. This is especially important for women (while also for men), given that the hospital system, especially when under stress of an epidemic, becomes more hierarchical and less human, reminding women of the depersonalization they have experienced in other aspects of their life in a society that has still not achieved gender equality and safety for women and girls. Last, it is important to celebrate the resilience of the human spirit, and how each individual draws upon the caring of those who love us (family members, the Universal Spirit of Love) to support ourselves through even the most dire, difficult moments that beset us.

Reflecting on Feminist Suggestions and the Practice of Medical Family Therapy: One Therapist's Personal Framework

Katherine M. Hertlein

Shannon came into my office for her weekly session, visibly shaken and upset. When I commented on her appearance, she reported that because she had difficulty managing her fibromyalgia over the week, it was difficult for her to get tasks accomplished around the house. Shannon felt alone and abandoned, as she had felt so many times in the past. Though I had spoken to Shannon about visiting her physician to gain more information on managing her fibromyalgia, she had yet to do so because she believed her physician thought she was exaggerating her symptoms and she feared being considered a hypochondriac.

Working to support Shannon pushed me to explore my personal framework for working with medical problems, particularly in cases with women in chronic conditions. As a student, I am still in the process of discovering who I am as a clinician. Though the ideas and thought processes presented here may not be entirely new, I am hopeful that presenting my journey to others will help them consider and develop their own framework for working with the intersection of gender issues and medical con-

Katherine M. Hertlein, MS, is a doctoral candidate in the Marriage and Family Therapy Program, Department of Human Development, Virginia Polytechnic Institute and State University, Blacksburg, VA 24061-0515.

[Haworth co-indexing entry note]: "Reflecting on Feminist Suggestions and the Practice of Medical Family Therapy: One Therapist's Personal Framework." Hertlein, Katherine M. Co-published simultaneously in *Journal of Feminist Family Therapy* (The Haworth Press, Inc.) Vol. 15, No. 2/3, 2003, pp. 127-136; and: *Feminist Perspectives in Medical Family Therapy* (ed: Anne M. Prouty Lyness) The Haworth Press, Inc., 2003, pp. 127-136. Single or multiple copies of this article are available for a fee from The Haworth Document Delivery Service [1-800-HAWORTH, 9:00 a.m. - 5:00 p.m. (EST). E-mail address: docdelivery@haworthpress.com].

cerns. Though this is just one voice, I am hopeful this will open the door to other conversations and other voices.

From my experience working with Shannon and other patients, it is clear that illness can have a profound effect on couples and families (Campbell & Patterson, 1995). Illness can create hardships and change how couples and families view themselves, their roles, and their capabilities. For example, in Shannon's case, she saw her role in the family as a homemaker and caretaker of her family. Also clear was that her illness affected her thoughts, behaviors, and interactions with others (consistent with Doyal's 1995 observations). Enduring fibromyalgia, particularly when it was difficult to manage, weighed on Shannon and depleted her of energy used to handle the stress of running a household. As a result, Shannon was often too exhausted to deal effectively with the stress in her life. She felt that her physician did not understand the effect that fibromyalgia had on her, leading her to feel abandoned. This isolation affected her socially and physically; Shannon would become depressed. Factors associated with an illness and its side effects may be not only difficult to deal with, but also be socially and physically problematic, potentially complicating overall functioning (Doyal, 1995).

Because illness and gender can be so intertwined, I felt that I needed to integrate health issues and gender issues into both individual and couple therapy. As a student, I had gained some exposure to medical family therapy and feminist thought, though not an integration of the two within a formal classroom setting. I had to rely on what I knew about feminist family therapy, medical family therapy, and my personal values to identify a framework that would work for me in practice.

INFUSING MEDICAL FAMILY THERAPY PRACTICE WITH FEMINIST IDEAS

I am at a point in my clinical development where I seek concrete interventions to assist me in treatment planning as well as opportunities to make theory my own. Realizing that I needed ideas about integrating feminist thoughts into agency and communion for Shannon, I inundated myself with information on how to best accomplish this. Specific techniques for employing feminist principles in family therapy have been organized under the principles of examination and making changes. Hare-Mustin (1978) established several techniques for family psychotherapists by providing a list of areas in which it is pertinent for a psychotherapist to intervene from a feminist-informed model of intervention;

Wilson (1993) challenged psychotherapists to understand the importance of gender in system organization. The gender metaframework provides a stand against oppression at all social levels, helping the family to recognize and work with gender constraints in their relationship (Breulin, Schwartz, & MacKune-Karrer, 1992); Mander and Rush (1974) identify feminist therapy freeing people from their restraining sex roles and becoming a whole person, including body therapy.

Yet of all of these, guidelines for conducting feminist family therapy that were most helpful to me at this time were those that provided a novice such as myself with a balance of concrete interventions and room for flexibility. Proposed by Walters, Carter, Papp, and Silverstein (1988), these methods also provide a place to examine the interaction between illness and relational systems. As a result of using a feminist lens, I have gained an additional awareness about gender differences in illness presentation, symptoms, and health care choices. Using a feminist lens extends the specialty of medical family therapy and pushes for gender- and culturally-sensitive interventions. Included in this summary are feminist family therapy themes that enable an explanation of traditional medical family therapy techniques: recognizing the biological dimension, soliciting the story, removing blame, maintaining communication, addressing developmental issues and agency, and leaving the door open for communication.

Looking at Agency and Communion Through a Feminist Lens

Agency. The two primary goals of medical family therapy, agency and communion, seemed to be consistent with the goals in Shannon's case. Agency refers to being an ambassador of one's own health by including a "sense of making personal choices in dealing with illness and the health care system, both of which often contribute to a patient's feeling of passivity and control" (McDaniel, Hepworth, & Doherty, 1992, p. 9). Patients are encouraged to commit to their health (Doherty, McDaniel, & Hepworth, 1994). For example, having a patient take charge of her health might include helping her learn to ask for support in managing diabetes from a family member, thus increasing agency. This was something that Shannon had struggled with from early on. Shannon and I had countless conversations regarding assertiveness in her health care decisions, and yet she was never able to quite commit to being assertive. Shannon believed that others would view her as demanding, impatient, and negative. I believed that this lack of assertiveness translated to Shannon as a lack of control. The less in control Shannon felt in her life, the more she felt depressed and alone. My goal, as her therapist, would be to facilitate a way in which she could feel her agency in her health care and encourage her assertiveness.

Medical family therapists, working to reduce an illness's power over a family, also empower patients (McDaniel et al., 1992). Incorporating the principle of *the personal is political* (Sturdivant, 1980) into medical family therapy allows patients to focus on external factors influencing their health care, reducing victim blame (also consistent with feminist empowerment strategies). Moving away from self-blame can help a patient adopt a more optimistic attitude. Medical family therapists who value the female perspective encourage agency by helping women to trust their intuition about medical problems and concerns, and support women in caring for their own needs and trusting their body experiences. In thinking about Shannon's case, she did not feel that she had any power in the relationship with her doctor, and made health care decisions based on how she feared being viewed rather than what was in her best interest. Personally, I could understand her concern: I, too, have often put off going to the doctor for what I viewed as a small concern, as to not appear too sensitive. This aspect, to benefit Shannon's overall well-being, was one focus of therapy.

Of the seven techniques presented in medical family therapy, there are several that are relevant to the integration of feminist family therapy and agency. In one technique, soliciting the illness story, the psychotherapist joins with the patient and his/her family (McDaniel et al., 1992). Through this process, I attempt to understand the family's history independent of the illness. This helps develop agency because the patient and I can identify strengths each present prior to the illness, and use these strengths throughout treatment to build agency. With a feminist-informed influence, I can solicit the illness story with a renewed emphasis on the role gender played throughout. In Shannon's case, gender may play a role in the communication about an illness in a family where men are taken more seriously than women, resulting in Shannon second-guessing herself. I had to be cognizant of this piece as Shannon and I worked, because it was important that Shannon knew I believed her. When a person has her decisions respected, she can feel more empowered and less vulnerable. I also believe that part of my role as a therapist is to assist patients to make informed decisions regarding their health care. When psychotherapists facilitate and support family decisions (rather than advise or direct), they encourage autonomy, confidence, and agency (McDaniel et al., 1992).

Communion. The second goal is communion, which aims to reunite the disabled or ill patient by reestablishing emotional bonds and support networks after the isolation of the illness or disability (Doherty et al., 1994; McDaniel, Hepworth, & Doherty, 1992; 1995). As illnesses move from the acute to the chronic phase, the ways in which partners or family members relate to each other change. Not all illnesses, however, follow the pattern of moving from acute to chronic. Some illnesses are intermittent and recurrent. Regardless of the course of the illness, communion is particularly important because when people can maintain communion with their family and social networks, they will likely receive more consistent support throughout the illness course, regardless of its pattern.

Communion is especially important because patients may feel isolated. I have experienced a lack of resources available in the community for patients with medical concerns, and usually have difficulty locating groups in the area for patients with medical concerns. I have often resorted to referring them to general groups such as those focusing on loss or grief, but patients often do not remain in the groups because of the lack of application. Awareness of communion as a critical factor in one's physical and emotional well-being made integrating communion of paramount importance when developing how I work with these cases. When the dyadic relationship of patients becomes more egalitarian, patients may feel more comfortable about approaching their partner when they need more support, meeting the goal of communion. Similarly, when a physician-patient relationship moves to be more egalitarian (somewhat flattening the hierarchy), patients may feel more comfortable approaching their physicians with questions and concerns, enhancing both agency and communion.

Be Aware of Societal Gender Messages and Gender Roles in Health Care

Awareness is key to providing feminist-informed therapy. It is critical that medical family therapists be aware that issues of gender can intersect with every aspect of patients' lives. For example, women are typically viewed as the nurturing individuals in a family relationship. In this role, women who are persistent about health concerns might be viewed as actively engaged in their caretaking role. As a result, female patients may believe physicians and/or psychotherapists do not take their concerns seriously and may attribute the nurturing stance of the physician or psychotherapist as insincere and merely a result of the job description rather than genuine interest.

Another important intervention in feminist-informed medical family therapy is the problem and/or response to illness with a particular emphasis on gender. For example, a woman with an illness such as diabetes mellitus may also experience feelings of sadness and uselessness because she does not have the ability to care for her family in the way she could in the past. She may be grieving the loss of her caretaking role as well as other losses that accompany her illness. A feminist-informed medical family therapist can normalize the feelings of grief and depression and place these feelings in a developmental context.

Gender-based differential treatment is an area of concern in the clinical setting (Stabb, Cox, & Harber, 1997). Biases have the potential to affect assessment and treatment strategies in many presenting problems. Reiker and Carmen (1984) support this assertion when they state: ". . . anger in women is often labeled as pathological rather than understood as a consequence of a devalued position" (p. 29). Women in therapy are also typically interrupted three times as much as men (Werner-Wilson, Price, Zimmerman, & Murphy, 1997). It is possible that this trend also occurs in the physician's office. Implications for differential treatment include adverse effects on a patient's sense of security, reduced comfort in asking questions, and refraining from inquiring about one's condition and options.

Acknowledgement of Fewer Resources for Women in Health Care

Women tend to have fewer resources than men in such aspects as society, psychotherapy, and medicine. Women also may be more vulnerable to certain disorders (Unger & Crawford, 1992). For example, lupus and fibromyalgia are more common in women than in men. As a result, resources should address the vulnerability of women to these disorders if they are to be adequate.

In a study by Phillips and Gilroy (1985), when psychotherapists identified characteristics of a healthy adult, these characteristics were no different than the picture of a healthy man. Yet the picture of a healthy woman, according to mental health practitioners, was different from the picture of a healthy man or a healthy adult (Broverman, Vogel, Broverman, Clarkson, & Rosenkrantz, 1972). Healthy women were considered more submissive, less dependent, less adventurous, more suggestive, less competitive, less illogical, and less objective. Implications of this study might be that men and women receive different treatment because there is a different picture of what an appropriate outcome would look like for men and women. This finding is consistent with what Shannon was feeling–that she would be viewed as illogical when presenting with a health complaint to her physician.

Psychotherapists recommend more medications and less therapy for elderly, depressed, female patients as opposed to younger women or men of any age (Ford & Sbordone, 1980; Ray, McKinney, & Ford, 1987). This might mean that psychotherapists view women as more pathological and needy of medical attention and medication. The result may be medications prescribed for women when they are not needed, or medications not prescribed for men when appropriate. Women receive twice as many prescriptions as men for psychotropic medications (Unger & Crawford, 1992). In general, women are given fewer options in medical care and are medicated more often than are men. Being aware of and acknowledging this phenomenon may help practitioners rethink prescribing medication for women. Psychotherapists can also understand how several medications, including psychotropic medications, may affect a patient's biological, psychological, and relational functioning. When Shannon and I discussed having her talk with her physician about medication options, she felt supported and ultimately more confident in making health care choices. If a woman is aware of the side effects of her medication and its influence on her biological, psychological, and relational functioning, she will be a better consumer of information regarding her health care, and employ decision-making that incorporates consideration of all of these aspects.

Address Unequal Power Distributions

Addressing unequal power distributions throughout treatment is critical to a feminist-informed medical family therapy model. Remaining open-minded about the potential influences of one's medical concerns includes an awareness of unequal power distributions, increased stress, how unequal power distributions affect a patient's daily functioning, and its influence on a patient's ability to comply with treatment protocols. The psychotherapist should listen carefully in the illness story and be sensitive to unequal power distributions in the telling of the story. McDaniel and her colleagues (1992) provide a list of questions to pose to the family to gain each member's perspective on the illness. The questions directed at family members of patients address how caring for the patient will be divided up among the family members. Feminist-informed psychotherapists should concern themselves with listening closely to the division of labor and pursue potential unequal power distributions.

Unequal power distributions may also occur in communication with patients. Two techniques, maintaining communication and leaving the door open for communication, are critical to the progression of therapy. Maintaining communication with physicians is crucial because it keeps the patient informed with diagnoses and treatment protocols. Unequal power distribution can affect communication between patients and their health care providers. For example, if a female patient believes she is treated differently because she is a woman, it may consequently affect how comfortable she feels about maintaining communication with her physician.

Establish a Relationship for Maintaining a Relationship with a Collaborative Health Care Team

Maintaining a relationship with the psychotherapist is also important. Patients should believe the psychotherapist is not providing differential care or giving power in the therapy to someone other than the patient due to one's gender. This may be difficult to accomplish when there is a serious health concern, as the patient will usually have someone assisting them with their care. Psychotherapists should examine their beliefs and actions in regard to giving power to men in the relationships, specifically if men are not the primary patients. Psychotherapists limit agency if they automatically place men in the "responsible" role without considering the larger message of their actions.

It is also essential for the psychotherapist to encourage communication between patients, physicians, and family members, engendering more comprehensive patient care (Walsh & Fortner, 2002). With adequate communication from physicians who have the ability to convey care and concern (Candib, 1995), patients feel "heard." In this safer environment, patients are more confident in conveying their needs for continuing medical and emotional care (Doherty et al., 1994; McDaniel et al., 1992). Within this safe zone, patients feel more secure and are able to better explore their environment. Patients like Shannon will explore options in their physical and emotional care, developing agency and communion. Encouraging Shannon to open the lines of communication between herself and her physician would help to increase her confidence in reporting her symptoms, and she would feel some element of a supportive network within the health care system.

Understanding the Medical Family Therapist's Role as a Social Agent

Just as medical family psychotherapists attempt to promote agency in the individual patients, psychotherapists must recognize they, too, are social agents and have a profound effect on patients. In the role of a social agent, a psychotherapist can be a significant model in promoting agency within the patient. In this manner, the psychotherapist and patient are collaborating to strengthen communion.

CONCLUSION

Feminist thought has informed many family therapy models and can be useful in expanding medical family therapy. Feminist-informed medical family therapy encourages psychotherapists to consider a larger systemic picture including engendered concepts of health and healing, and the integration of feminist family therapy and medical family therapy provides a lens in which medical family therapists can view and treat cases through a feminist framework. Integrating both feminist and medical family therapy is important because it provides more comprehensive care to women, men, and families, resulting in gender-sensitive treatment. In Shannon's case, when we were able to identify the factors that prevented her from developing agency and communion, we were able to set more specific goals and work through the constraints. Shannon eventually felt confident to assert herself and talk about options with her physician. Once she began communicating with her physician, she reported that her husband began to take time to listen to her concerns and work toward further role flexibility within their couple relationship.

Though this article is just the beginning, I hope that my development within these pages assists others who are struggling with the integration of feminism in medical family therapy. Patients who feel vulnerable within the medical arena can benefit significantly from a therapy that incorporates agency and communion while considering how gender influences their ability to employ agency and communion in their lives. Future work might include building on the themes presented and moving toward an expanded feminist-informed medical family therapy framework. Elements of an expanded framework might include specific medical family therapy interventions that consider gender as a factor in patients' lives, further interventions that are sensitive to cultural idiosyncrasies and those which incorporate agency and communion in a gender-sensitive way with all family members.

REFERENCES

Breunlin, D., Schwartz, R., & MacKune-Karrer, B. (1992). *Metaframeworks: Transcending the models of family therapy.* San Francisco, CA: Jossey-Bass.
Broverman, I. K., Vogel, S. R., Broverman, D. M., Clarkson, F. E., & Rosenkrantz, P. S. (1972). Sex-role stereotypes: A current appraisal. *Journal of Social Issues, 28*(2), 59-78.

Campbell, T. L., & Patterson, J. M. (1995). The effectiveness of family interventions in the treatment of physical illness. *Journal of Marital and Family Therapy, 21*(4), 545-583.

Candib, L. M. (1995). *Medicine and the family: A feminist perspective.* New York: Basic Books.

Doherty, W. J., McDaniel, S. H., & Hepworth, J. (1994). Medical family therapy: An emerging arena for family therapy. *Journal of Family Therapy, 16*(1), 31-46.

Doyal, L. (1995). *What makes women sick.* New Brunswick, NJ: Rutgers University.

Ford, C. V., & Sbordone, R. J. (1980). Attitudes of psychiatrists toward elderly patients. *American Journal of Psychiatry, 137*, 571-575.

Hare-Mustin, R. T. (1978). A feminist approach to family therapy. *Family Process, 17*, 181-194.

Mander, A. V., & Rush, A. K. (1974). *Feminism as therapy.* New York: Random House.

McDaniel, S. H., Hepworth, J. L., & Doherty, W. J. (1995). Medical family therapy with somaticizing patients: The co-creation of therapeutic stories. *Family Process, 34*, 349-361.

McDaniel, S. H., Hepworth, J., & Doherty, W. J. (1992). *Medical family therapy.* New York: Basic Books.

Phillips, R. D., & Gilroy, F. D. (1985). Sex-role stereotypes and clinical judgments of mental health: The Brovermans' findings reexamined. *Sex Roles, 12*, 179-193.

Ray, D. C., McKinney, K. A., & Ford, C. V. (1987). Ageism in psychiatrists: Associations with gender, certification, and theoretical orientation. *The Gerontologist, 27*, 82-86.

Reiker, P. P., & Carmen, E. (1984). *The gender gap in psychotherapy.* New York: Plenum.

Stabb, S. D., Cox, D. L., & Harber, J. L. (1997). Gender-related therapist attributions in couples therapy: A preliminary multiple case study investigation. *Journal of Marital and Family Therapy, 23*(3), 335-346.

Sturdivant, S. (1980). *Therapy with women.* New York: Springer Publishing Company.

Unger, R., & Crawford, M. (1992). *Women and gender: A feminist psychology.* New York: McGraw Hill.

Walsh, S. R., & Fortner, J. (2002). Coming full circle: Family therapy and psychiatry reunite in a training program. *Families, Systems & Health, 20*, 105-111.

Walters, M., Carter, B., Papp, P., & Silverstein, O. (1988). *The invisible web.* New York: Guilford.

Werner-Wilson, R. J., Price, S. J., Zimmerman, T. S., & Murphy, M. J. (1997). Client gender as a process variable in marriage and family therapy: Are women clients interrupted more than men clients? *Journal of Family Psychology, 11*, 373-377.

Wilson, R. J. (1993). Differential treatment of men and women in marriage and family therapy. Unpublished doctoral dissertation. University of Georgia.

Index

The letter "n" in italics indicates notes.

ACTH (adrenocorticotropic hormone), 12
Adrenocorticotropic hormone (ACTH), 12
Agency issues
  cancer and family life cycle, 102, 103,107-108,109,110,111, 113,115
  feminist medical family therapy perspective on, 129-130
  patient power over illness, 130
  social agent role of therapist, 134-135
American Academy of Family Physicians, 78
Anxiety disorders, 2

Behavioral science training, in family medicine, 60-62,
  behavioral health clinic case example, 81-86,86n. 2
  gender and biology focus
    clinical implications, 17-18
    emotion, importance of, 3-5
    empowering women, 18
    genetic indeterminism, 8-10
    multilevel feedback framework, 10-12,11fig.
    nature vs. nurture issue, 2-3
    nurturing relationships and health, 5-7
    plasticity of the brain, 7-8
    summary regarding, 1,18-19
Being-in-relation approach to clinical relationship, 58-59,69-70
Biopsychosocial model of healing, 61, 67-70

collaborative care, 80
mind-body-spirit connection, xiii
vulvar vestibulitis syndrome, 95
Bischof, Gary H., 23
Brain plasticity, 7-8

Cancer. See Gender roles, family life cycle, and cancer
Collaboration
  gender and power issues in, 24-27
  See also Collaborative care in family medicine; Power and gender issues in collaborative relationships
Collaborative care in family medicine
  behavioral health clinic case example, 81-86,86n. 2
  biopsychosocial systems model, 80
  family medicine culture, 77-79
  joint training, 80-81, 86n. 1
  mental health services focus, 76-79
  physician and therapist collaboration, 79-80
  Somatoform Disorder, 85
  summary regarding, 75-76,86
Communion issues
  cancer and family life cycles, 102, 103,107-108,109,110,113, 115
  in chronic illnesses, 131
  social agent role of therapist, 135
Confidentiality, 40-41
Connected knowing, 59-60,63-64
  empathy and, 65
Connor, Jennifer, 89
Cortical-releasing hormone (CRH), 12
Couples therapy. See Vulvar vestibulitis syndrome, couples therapy

For Product Safety Concerns and Information please contact our
EU representative GPSR@taylorandfrancis.com Taylor & Francis
Verlag GmbH, Kaufingerstraße 24, 80331 München, Germany